MW01265306

Lose the Diet

*Transform your
body by connecting
with your soul*

KATHY BALLAND

LOSE THE DIET
Kathy Balland

Published by: Blissful Publications, LLC
                    3116 S. Mill Avenue #429
                    Tempe, AZ 85282

Web site: www.LoseTheDiet.com

Copyright © 2009 by Blissful Publications

All rights reserved. No part of this book may be reproduced or transmitted in any form or by any means, electronic or mechanical, including photocopying, recording, or via any information storage and retrieval system without written permission from the author, except for the inclusion of brief quotations in a review.

Printed in the United States of America
10 9 8 7 6 5 4 3 2 1

Library of Congress Control Number: 2008909580
ISBN: 978-0-9821831-0-6

Disclaimer

Every effort has been made to make this book as complete and as accurate as possible. However, there may be mistakes both typographical and in content. Therefore, this text should be used only as a general guide.

The purpose of this book is to educate. The author shall have neither liability nor responsibility to any person or entity with respect to any loss or damage caused, directly or indirectly by the information contained in this book.

Page production by One-On-One Book Production, West Hills, CA

This book is dedicated to all of those beautiful souls who are weary of the dieting yo-yo. May you reconnect with yourself and discover the power within you for health and happiness.

Acknowledgments

$\mathcal{I}$ would like to thank the following people, whose connection with me has allowed me to connect with my true self.

Mary Cornell: A life coach who goes "beyond" the norm.

K.C. Miller: For your inspiration and being the catalyst to launch a million dreams.

Linda Bennett: For opening peoples hearts and minds, and providing tools so that we can assist others in their healing.

Thanks to **Elise** for the continued insight, and to **Lena** for always listening.

To dad: For keeping the connection, and in the most unexpected ways.

To mom: For providing unending support and encouragement.

Thanks to **Louise Hay, Marci Shimoff, Deepak Chopra, Mark Victor Hansen, Jack Canfield** and the many great authors and speakers who enrich our daily lives.

And finally, many thanks to **Richard** — My Rock of Cachel.

TABLE OF CONTENTS

Introduction

As a Mind-Body Wellness Practicioner, I have studied the mind-body-soul connection, and how our thoughts and feelings ultimately affect our well-being. And as I observed what was going on from day to day, I began to see the insanity of the weight issue in our society. (As Albert Einstein said, insanity is doing the same thing over and over and expecting different results.) In the world of hypnotherapy I came to realize the number one issue that people want help with is weight.

When I dug deeper into the weight issue, I began to put the pieces of the puzzle together. Certainly self-esteem is a valid reason for the weight imbalance, and that has to do with the loss of connection with ourselves. I also observed that people can feel disconnected from others, and they may attempt to fill that emptiness with food. And finally, there can be a loss of connection from our higher self, or God.

As I looked back on my own experiences, I could see how they affected me; mentally, emotionally, and physically. There were times when I had

1

struggled with my own self-esteem, as I experienced the divorce of my parents, as well as my own divorce. For years I tried to reconnect with my father, who had distanced himself. (He was an alcoholic.) And as I struggled to do so, I became involved in unhealthy relationships, in my attempt fulfill the connection I had lost.

During my unhappy marriage, I gained a few too many pounds, as I attempted to stay in what was a miserable situation. My fear of being alone drove me to convince myself that at least I had "someone." That is why I stuffed my unhappy emotions with food.

I slowly began to realized that I needed to first love myself before I could truly love anyone else, and that healthy relationships needed to be a give-and-take situation which is part of loving ourselves. Upon that realization, I found a healthy balance in my life by connecting the mental, emotional and physical level.

When my father passed away, I felt a terrible loss even though it had been many years since I had actually seen my father, the finality of losing him seemed devastating because I had lost the hope of re-connecting with him.

In the year following his death, I slowed down, and my metabolism slowed down as well.

As I ate to "feel better," I once again put on some weight. But as I healed my emotions and sense of loss, partly by connecting with others, I once again found balance.

Along the way, I searched for other clues to the huge weight imbalance in our society, and in my quest, I have discovered certain tools to help people to not only achieve a healthy weight, but to also maintain a healthy weight. My goal is to restore sanity in our "disconnected" society, so that we can live healthy, happy and prosperous lives.

Living a healthy life is very important, everyone knows that, but knowing and doing are two different things. For me I knew I needed to be better but it took me a long time to find my path to getting there. Three years ago I began a journey that resulted in losing 65 pounds. I went from a size 22, 24 to a size 14 today. I had begun my weight loss journey when I had my first session with Kathy. I am an emotional, stress eater and found my session with Kathy to be very relaxing. It allowed me to work towards my continuing weight loss goals. During our first season and additional discussions I found Kathy to be very knowledgeable about weight loss and the reasons why people over eat. It has been a joy to work with Kathy and gain from her knowledge and experience!

Thanks for everything Kathy!
Christi Hohensee

1

What's Going On?

Now there are more overweight people in America than average-weight people. So overweight people are now average. Which means you've met your New Year's resolution.

– Jay Leno

If you look at today's society, you'll become aware of how overweight people have generally become. From talk shows to news programs, weight is a constant topic. Obesity has continued to be on the rise, becoming one of the main threats to health. The Obesity Action Coalition reports that obesity impacts one in four Americans. It is estimated that more than 93 million Americans are obese, and that number is predicted to increase to 120 million in the next five years.

The resulting healthcare costs are enormous (in the hundreds of billions). But why is there increasing obesity when there are more diet books and programs on the market every day? There is a ton (excuse the pun) of information out there. But, why isn't it working?

Dieting people are focused on the numbers — the pounds, calories, carbs, fat grams, etc. obesity still seems to be a problem. Maybe it is time to lose the diet and throw away the scale and forget the numbers. The obsession with numbers is not really controlling the weight problem instead it is a loss of control.

Our ancestors weren't aware or worried about carbs and fat intake. They ate what they wanted and it generally was a good square meal. They did not analyze the foods that were available as so many of us do today. With all the dietary studies, we know much more about food than our ancestors did. It is now mandatory to label all the ingredients in the packaged foods we buy. The one exception, of course, the produce department — where foods are in their natural form. With all this knowledge — the reading of labels — learning what is best for us to eat — obesity rates continue to climb.

It has been proven to me that the answer to obesity is much deeper than our layers of fat (or the lack of). The answer is much more effective than all the numbers that we calculate and read on our bathroom scale. We must look into our soul; into our inner being for the key to the weight problem. We need to connect with our mind, body and soul, not just flesh, bones and muscle mass.

Take a look at all of the diet-oriented food out there. There is low-fat, no-fat, sugar-free and low carb. What have we got left? Some people seem to think the answer is a few leaves, nuts and twigs. Yet society, as a whole, is getting heavier from this continuing attempt at deprivation (diet), which just causes a yo-yo effect of weight loss followed by weight gain.

Eating Disorders

Then there are eating disorders such as binge-eating, where people eat large quantities of food in a short period of time, while feeling out of control. There is muscle dysmorphia. This is caused by men who work out to excess, while consuming large amounts of protein to build a bigger body. They may even resort to steroids. Yet, they never seem to feel adequate as they continue on their relentless quest to obtain even bigger muscles.

At the other end of the spectrum are the anorexics and bulemics. Those people who try desperately to maintain an abnormally low weight. They may not realize that they are slowly starving themselves to the point of non-existence, either by not eating enough food, or by binge-eating and purging.

Also, there are women who take "staying in shape" to extremes. They, too, maintain a dangerously low body weight, as they virtually exercise themselves to death. Like anorexia, their body becomes so out of balance that they are no longer menstruating. This disorder is known as "female athlete syndrome."

The amazing fact about these eating disorders, where people maintain a dangerously low weight, only exists in industrialized nations, and most particularly in the U.S. In less developed countries, people do not seem to have the need to starve themselves. So, why is there such an imbalance in our society? What's going on?

There are many things that are used or done to excess in today's world. The emptiness that is felt from the stress and strain that our modern lifestyle creates has resulted in people trying to fill their emptiness in various ways. From drugs and alcohol to credit card abuse and living beyond our means, while trying to satisfy our soul with food. However, the emptiness still remains.

As I mentioned before, too often people are focused on the number of calories, grams, exchanges and various calculations — a mechanical process. They check out the percentages, ratios and the body mass index (which does not take into account certain variables such as bone density and muscle mass). After all, we are all built differently.

Don't Compare Yourself with the Stars

Then there is the scale, which is just another set of numbers in the seemingly endless parade of calculations. Women in particular become obsessed with the need to be at the "perfect" weight and look like women in magazine ads. No matter how hard anyone tries it never seems good enough. In today's society, we are bombarded with images of stick-thin people. How realistic is that? Or more to the point, how healthy is that?

As you look at the actors and actresses who have the "perfect" bodies, be aware that those people have personal trainers and chefs who help them on a day-to-day basis to maintain that level of fitness. In fact, there was an article in which a famous actress admitted that it was not fair to the average person to compare themselves to her, since she had the time and money to invest in her appearance.

And don't forget that many of the photos of the stars and models we see are artificially enhanced. This adds to the misperception that we can achieve that look. We should strive for health and fitness, but we can all drive ourselves crazy by trying to emulate the perfect air-brushed photos.

Unfortunately, some people go overboard trying to duplicate the image of a perfect body, and the result can be ill health. What usually happens is we begin dieting and yo-yo through life as we keep fighting to lower our weight — and then gain even more pounds back when we revert back to the same old eating habits after slowing down our metabolism.

Connecting with our Higher Power

The fact is that today most of us have lost connection — the connection with ourselves, our inner power and with other people. When the body is treated as a separate system from our mind and our soul, then permanent weight change cannot occur. Typically, the attitude of Western science has been that our inner being is independent from our bodies, that is certainly one of the reasons obesity continues to be an issue.

Our fast-paced lifestyle has had a negative affect on people's weight. It's not just "keeping up with the Joneses" — today's economy forces both mom and dad into the work force — this separates them from their family, friends and a sense of community, leaving them feeling unfulfilled. They have a sense of emptiness. This can create the need to fill up with food, then diet — starting a cycle of loss and gain.

A better solution is to create time in which to reconnect to ourselves, our family and other people. We must choose to re-connect, and find the love and positive energy that will allow us to feel satisfied from our body to our soul. By connecting with the mind, soul and body, we can maintain a better balance for health and well being.

Maybe There Is Hope

Perhaps our society is beginning to see the light. Nowadays, even bariatric specialists (doctors who treat people for obesity) are beginning to approach obesity from various fronts, understanding that there is a mind-body connection. Physicians are now working with patients to learn about their motivations and values. They may discuss self-nurturing habits and healthy new routines, and help to create an attitude that maximizes the mind- body connection.

I want to show you how you can make the mind-body-soul connection. In the following chapters I will offer insight and suggestions that have been effective, and have given people a choice — a choice to live more healthy lives while enjoying the food they eat.

2

Die-it

I've been on a diet for two weeks and all I've lost is two weeks.

– Totie Fields

*B*roken into two syllables, the word Die-it is enough to send chills up the spines of those who know what it is like to deprive themselves without getting long-term results. In some cases there may be immediate results (especially in the case of losing water weight), but in the long run, the weight can come back (and then some).

After all, if you completely deprive yourself of the foods you love, are you really living the life you deserve? Are you savoring all of the wonderful flavors that food has to offer? We are not living this life to starve ourselves, but to nourish ourselves. We are meant to enjoy the smells, textures and flavors of foods, and to appreciate the rich diversity of the cultural differences in food. As the character Auntie Mame said "life is a banquet."

Why Diets Don't Work

There have been thousands of diets, yet there has not been one diet that ultimately works because, for one thing, it is not possible to maintain someone else's way of eating. If you grew up eating your family's ethnic food, and now, you are not allowed to eat that food because it is not on some diet plan, you are not being true to yourself. It doesn't feel right, because the diet is not about who you really are. There is a sense of a loss of identity, and eventually you must go off of the diet to return to "homeostasis" or your true self.

"Dieting" can actually trigger us to overeat. We can become overly focused on not allowing ourselves to have food by saying things like "I want that, but I can't eat it." In the end, we wind up wanting it even more because of feeling so deprived. When we suddenly allow ourselves to eat the "forbidden" food, we usually indulge because it is so special to us. It tastes so good we gorge ourselves and end up back where we started.

Certain foods can be labeled "good" or "bad," causing us to place a value judgment on them. But food is neither good or bad, it is simply food. However, if we eat what we see as "bad" food, we feel ashamed of ourselves, which hurts our self-esteem. So why do that? Are we not entitled to taste those foods now and then? If you "beat yourself up" for eating the forbidden food, then you may want to really binge, and the vicious negative cycle of "bad" food and feeling like a "bad" person spirals out of control.

When we stop denying ourselves foods we enjoy, we can stop feeling deprived. We should realize that it is acceptable to taste the foods that we love, and eat those foods without feeling guilty. We, then, won't feel the need to binge. We can choose to eat a modest amount and really taste and enjoy. We can find a good balance by respecting ourselves and our choices.

The True Issue Behind Obesity

So many people are looking at weight from a physical perspective. The issue of weight has to do with the underlying reality behind the weight "imbalance" in our society. The use of food is really a by-product of what is going on inside of us. In other words, it's about what is going on *inside* (such as our habits and emotions), not what's on the *outside*. If a person only looks at weight from the standpoint of food, they are not getting to the root of their real problem, and the excess weight will most likely return.

In addition, losing weight from the outside in is very mechanical. When it comes to counting calories and calculating, it's all about the numbers. However, people are not made of numbers. They have emotions, hearts and souls. And, it's time to stop searching out "there" — calories, the scale, diet foods or gimmicks, because the answer to the weight issue cannot be found outside of ourselves.

Consuming pre-packaged diet foods may give a person instant gratification as they begin to lose the weight. However, once the pre-packaged food is gone, the person's body can easily revert to the way it was. After all, the person who is on the diet is not preparing the food themselves, and, therefore, is not learning a permanent way to balance one's weight. When the special diet food is taken away, it can be very difficult to maintain the achieved weight. Any emotional eating that was previously there, can easily come back again.

No Magic Pill or Fad Diets

There are advertisements that offer the "easy way out" with a "magic" diet pill. This may be tempting, but it does not deal with the underlying issues, and these pills can cause permanent physical problems, such as heart damage. In the end, the diet pills do not appear to be a healthy or permanent choice in weight management. Even if we look at weight from a physical perspective, diets still do not work. So many fad diets cut out entire food groups, (which isn't healthy) and require us to deprive ourselves of the foods we love.

Fat is Stored Energy

Understand, fat is not necessarily a bad word. Fat is simply stored energy. In fact, fat is essential to the body (like essential fatty acids.) Fat is actually needed to absorb certain nutrients. When people go "overboard" in their quest to slim down, they actually defeat their purpose. In fact, many prescribed diets do not provide *enough* calories for effective weight loss.

Sometimes people try fasting, however only about half of the weight that they lose while fasting is actually fat. In fact, weight loss from fasting can be described as a reduction of the total body weight, due to a mean loss of fluid, body fat or adipose tissue and/or lean mass, namely bone mineral deposits, muscle, tendon and other connective tissue.

If we lose muscle from "under" eating, our bodies burn less fat, even when we are simply sitting still. Five pounds of muscle burns about 200 calories per day, without doing any exercise. So, under eating can defeat the whole purpose of reducing the amount of fat in our bodies.

The reality is that you should never eat less than 10 times your ideal body weight in calories. For example, 150 pounds would be 1500 calories per day. If you eat less than that, after a period of time your body will slow down the burning of fat in order to survive. The scary thing is when people diet, they are often not consuming *enough* calories to maintain a healthy body. When people go overboard with dieting and over-training, it actually *slows down* their metabolism. It is much better to free yourself from a vicious cycle of deprivation.

A healthy body fat range for men is 10 to 15 percent. Women should have at least 15 percent body fat in order to maintain a normal menstrual cycle. Too little fat changes hormone levels, which can result in the loss of bone mass (and osteoporosis). Also, the lack of menstruation results in the stagnation of tissue in the uterus, and can lead to cysts and tumors.

The truth is that a person who weighs 180 pounds is able to eat more calories to get down to 120 pounds, than a 130-pound person can eat to get down to 120 pounds. Generally, a heavier person can eat more food than they think in order to lose weight. So assuming that you are not eating enough, if you increase your food intake, you can increase your body's capacity to burn energy, and ultimately lose weight. Just think of eating food like putting wood on a fire. If you don't put enough wood on the fire, then the fire cannot burn.

Here's a thought: Does someone who appears to be at a healthy weight count calories? Just ask them. The answer will probably be "NO." But if you still want an idea of how many calories you can (or should) consume to reach and maintain a particular weight, the following is a "rule of thumb."

If your ideal weight is 150 pounds, you would start by multiplying it by 10 to get 1500 calories (which is the basic amount needed for burning energy). Add another third of that (500 calories) for total energy expenditure, or the additional calories needed for normal physical activity. Add that together to get 2,000 calories, and add an additional 10 percent of that (200 calories) which your body needs to metabolize food. The grand total would be 2,200 calories per day, which may be more than you thought.

> **To put it more simply: 1,500 + 500 (1/3rd) = 2,000 + 200 (10%) = 2,200**

So if your ideal weight is higher than 150 pounds, then you can consume even more calories to achieve that weight. But who wants to count calories? Calorie counting is not exactly fun, and who has the time anyway? Let's talk about a more sensible approach, which includes various key elements to weight management.

The Right Way to Eat

So, how do you eat to burn the fat? Eating regularly has a tendency to keep the metabolism going. Skipping breakfast is not recommended. If breakfast is skipped, then it puts the body in fasting mode, which slows down the metabolism. (That is why they call it break-fast.)

The problem with fasting is the body has a tendency to think there is a famine going on, and it begins to find ways to store fat (in case of an emergency). It does this by making a genesis enzyme that causes the fat to sort of "stick together," so that it stays in the fat cell, and does not get released into the blood stream. If it is not released into the bloodstream, then it cannot be used as energy. Starvation and deprivation are no help in winning the weight battle.

To stop the vicious cycle, try spreading your meals out. It is also better than eating too much at once, because if you consume too much in one sitting, it results in the storage of more fat. Several smaller meals (like five per day) is a better way to keep the metabolism going. In other words, snacking isn't such a bad thing. If your stomach is growling and you feel hungry, it is better to put something in it to keep the metabolism going. And, you never feel deprived. Isn't that great?

Of course, snacking with whole foods is the best way to go. (A Twinkie is not a whole food.) Eat foods like fruit, nuts (in moderation) a cheese stick, or anything that is relatively natural that you would enjoy. You know, the way nature intended. Some people snack on a few walnuts, which can help you feel full, especially when you eat them before a meal. That can also help prevent over-indulging.

Whole foods are better for you than processed foods that are man made. The processed foods usually contain sugar and corn syrup. It's amazing what they put these sweeteners in. (Why do we need sweetener in condiments like ketchup and tartar sauce?) However, there are some brands that do not use sweeteners.

For example, many stores carry a natural peanut butter that does not contain sweeteners. If you can avoid those unnecessary additives, your body will thank you. And, you will feel just as full, and you won't even miss it, because you are still eating a satisfying quantity of food rather than cutting out food.

By simply checking the labels and choosing brands that do not contain (or are low in) sugar or corn syrup, can do your body a favor by giving it something that is healthier. (Not to mention that sugary ingredients can also lead to cravings.) Once you learn which foods are best, you can make a habit of making healthier choices.

Besides food, there is the often over-looked area of what we drink. Reducing our intake of sugary beverages alone can decrease sugar cravings that can cause us to over-indulge.

Some diets recommend very low or no carbohydrates. However, carbohydrates are not a bad thing, especially the complex carbs that are in fruits, vegetables and *whole* grains. Some examples are: Whole grain breads, oats and brown rice. Complex carbohydrates can actually help you to feel full longer, because they are broken down into glucose more slowly than simple (sugary) carbs. The result is a steady stream of energy throughout the day. Again, the more natural (or whole) the food is, the less refined sugar there tends to be. Focus on food quality instead of food quantity.

Some women have a problem with water retention, and what may appear to be fat is actually excess water in the body. Sometimes excess water occurs with increased estrogen levels. There are various natural ways to reduce water retention.

For example, there are various *whole* foods than can help counteract water retention, such as bananas. The potassium in bananas can reduce fluid retention. Cabbage is a natural diuretic, and you can eat it as coleslaw, in a salad, or in a sandwich. Cranberry juice is also recommended to reduce water retention (preferably the kind without a lot of added sugar). Vitamins A and C can help reduce water retention. And, if you have overeaten and feel bloated, you can eat some plain low fat yogurt with active cultures to aid in digestion.

How to Eat

When you eat, pay attention to what you are eating. It is best to sit down, relax and enjoy your food by eating slowly and appreciating each bite.

Notice how you feel when you are eating. Are you enjoying the taste and texture of the food? Keep in mind that it takes about 20 minutes for the brain to realize that the stomach is full. By eating too quickly, the message will come too late, and you will already have been full for awhile, maybe to the point of being "stuffed." In this case, the phrase "go with your gut" has new meaning.

You don't have to follow all of the eating "rules" all of the time. The point is to be aware of how the body uses food, so that you can make adjustments that work for you. Then, hopefully you can prevent the yo-yo syndrome of losing excess fat and putting it back on. After all, this constant dramatic weight gain and weight loss puts more stress on the body than a person who remains at an unhealthy weight. The key is to gradually reach a healthy weight and maintain it without too much fluctuation.

Above all, diets miss the point when it comes to the relationship between the mind, body and soul. No matter what diet a person is on, if they eat habitually or emotionally, their weight can get out of control. But, the person has a choice — they can choose to get connected — mind, body and soul, by using a few useful tools which are

given in the following chapters in order to
achieve and maintain a healthy weight

3

How Sweet It Is

Sham Harga had run a successful eatery for many years by always smiling, never extending credit, and realizing that most of his customers wanted meals properly balanced between the four food groups: Sugar, starch, grease, and burnt crunchy bits.

– Terry Pratchett, Men at Arms

When people lose a sense of connection, they can begin to fill the emptiness with whatever they think will help satisfy their soul. The large quantity of sweets that many people consume is only a temporary "fix" to fill the emptiness. Over time, too many sweets can become a habit, and ultimately, an addiction. Not to mention the health consequences of over-indulging in sweets.

Today, sugar is being used for self-medication. For instance, sweets are used when a person is lacking energy or they are trying to improve their mood. People often deny that they have a sugar "addiction" and this is similar to a drug addiction. If they don't have their sugary or processed foods at different intervals throughout the day (like at each meal, or between each meal), they may find themselves getting irritable. Does this sound like you? Be honest with yourself — become aware.

All about Sugar

Sugar is a refined chemical. It is harvested from sugarcane, then refined just like opium is refined from poppies, and cocaine is refined from coca leaves. We know that the more processed a food is, the less nutritive value it has, and since sugar is refined at least six times, it has little if any nutritive value. It's amazing how something changes when you take it out of nature, and alter its natural form. This man-made substance (sugar) can be turned into substance-abuse, when it is used like a drug. Enjoying a good piece of chocolate can be compared to a person who enjoys a fine glass of wine. However, when sweets are abused, they become dangerous to a person's health and well-being.

While we are busy fighting drug abuse, taxpayer dollars are subsidizing the sugar industry. Perhaps it has to do with the fact that so many people are addicted to it, and the sugar industry is backed by a powerful political lobby. Because of this, refined white sugar is inexpensive and available to everyone in the country. And, it has become a common recreational drug. The pleasurable affects of sugar makes it what is commonly known as a "comfort food." When it is used in excess, sugar is considered to be more dangerous to the human body than marijuana, and it is more addictive than cocaine.

Sugar is probably the most common drug there is. America and other western cultures have become addicted to not only sugar, but other sweeteners such as corn syrup. The use of corn syrup or HFCS (high fructose corn syrup) has become a staple in the American diet by being added to a huge amount of processed foods.

These sweet substances are not just in the most obvious foods such as cookies, but also put in canned fruits and vegetables, peanut butter, ketchup, bread, yogurt, cereal, salad dressing, spaghetti sauce, and in just about every processed food there is. Prove it to yourself. Check the labels. You will see just how many sweeteners are added to almost everything.

According to the USDA, sweetened fruit drinks account for 10 percent of the added sugars that are consumed. Candy and cake each contribute five percent of the sugar. Breakfast cereal, table sugar, honey, cookies, brownies, syrups and toppings each comprise four percent of the added sugars that are eaten. The average American ingests 32 teaspoons of refined sugar per day. This refined sugar is not really a food, it is a chemical.

The biochemical qualities of white sugar are almost identical to alcohol except for one molecule. But unlike alcohol or drugs, sugar is viewed as an acceptable addiction rather than a serious health problem. Besides the depletion of vitamins and minerals, some of the symptoms of excessive sugar consumption include: anxiety, depression, irritability, hyperactivity, panic attacks, adrenal fatigue, candida overgrowth, tooth decay, hyperactivity, chromium deficiency, type II diabetes, hypoglycemia, raised cholesterol levels, mood swings and behavioral problems.

The Effects of Too Much Sugar

Consuming too much sugar can also lead to: A loss of tissue elasticity and altering the structure of collagen which can cause pre-mature aging, weakened eyesight, problems with the digestive tract, alcoholism, gallstones, appendicitis, hemorrhoids, varicose veins, osteoporosis, food allergies, cardiovascular disease, toxemia during pregnancy, cataracts and nearsightedness, emphysema, Parkinson's disease, damage to the pancreas, increased fluid retention, migraines, increased risk of gout, Alzheimer's disease and hormone imbalances.

When it comes to weight management, the body metabolizes sugar into two to five times more fat than it does with starch. And, obese people can experience high blood pressure from excessive amounts of sugar. Sugar also suppresses the immune system, by depleting the levels of phagocytes, or white blood cells, which are required for immune function. These cells also destroy harmful bacteria. The loss of the white blood cells cuts down on the body's ability to fight disease and infection.

Sugary foods can actually affect the brain like cocaine, and research has discovered that rats will choose sugar water over cocaine. (The sugar water has more of a reward affect on the brain than cocaine.) The lab rats developed sugar dependence over a period of 10 days.

Sugar addiction can trigger withdrawal symptoms that resemble drug addiction, and can include anxiety, chattering teeth and tremors. Even when the sugar is replaced with artificial sweeteners, there is a similar behavior. The excessive amount of sweet taste creates the sugar dependence.

"Added" Sugar in Our Foods

Although it may be virtually impossible to cut out sugar completely, it is possible to at least keep sugar consumption balanced. After all, the amount of sugary ingredients or sweeteners that the average American consumes overall has at one point reached an all-time high of 158.4 pounds per year. That's just under ½ pound per day. The breakdown of the sweeteners is:

> 89.1 pounds of corn sweeteners
> 67.9 pounds of cane and beet sugars
> 1.4 pounds of other sugars

This is just "added" sugar, which does not include natural sugars in milk, fruit and vegetables, which people should be consuming more of because of the nutrients in those foods. Also, the difference between fructose or natural sugar in fruit versus processed sugars, is that fructose still has its chemical bonds intact.

Because of these chemical bonds, it takes longer for the body to break down the natural sugar. Over time, the amount of sugar that is released is more moderate. The energy boost from fruit is more gradual, and the mood is slightly elevated rather than becoming suddenly elevated.

It should be mentioned that low fat foods are generally high in sugar. For example, fat-free or low-fat salad dressing can be high in sugar, as the fat is replaced with sweeteners. Although it may say low fat, it can still be high in calories.

In 1986, the U.S. Food and Drug Administration predicted that sugar consumption would level off and decline in the next few years, but that did not happen. Instead, it is estimated that 25 percent of supermarket aisle space is used for sugary foods. Also, just because a product says "natural," doesn't mean that it does not contain high-fructose corn syrup. That's because the Food and Drug Administration never established rules on what "natural" means.

Since 1960, corn and other caloric sweeteners have become more heavily used, and are a staple in the American diet. The use of corn syrup came about in the 1960s when the corn market prices declined, resulting in commodity prices failing to cover the costs of production for farmers. When that happened, government subsidies became important.

Corn syrup was developed since it has a longer shelf life and is inexpensive to produce.

With the advent of corn syrup, farmers were still able to receive corn subsidies, and processed food became less expensive to produce. With the consumption of all of the processed and convenience food, Americans began consuming too much added sugar.

It is recommended that a person who eats 2,200 calories per day should consume a maximum amount of 12 teaspoons of added sugar, which is a little more than a can of soda.

Soft Drinks

And soft drinks are probably the largest source of sugar in the American diet. There is almost one pound of refined sugar in each gallon of soft drink, or 10 teaspoons per 12 ounce can. In 1999, 39.1 gallons of soft drinks were consumed by each person. That's about one fourth of the amount of sweetener that is consumed by each person, each year.

By 2003, Americans were drinking 46 gallons of soft drinks, or four times the amount (11 gallons) that were consumed in 1950. It is clear that cutting down on sweetened beverages can have a big impact on obesity.

Dessert for Breakfast

Another issue is that the American diet consists of what other countries would call dessert for breakfast. The high-sugar and/or high-fat content of foods such as donuts, danishes, muffins, pancakes and waffles with syrup, not to mention sugary cereals, is not a very healthy way to start the day and get the metabolism going.

A better choice for breakfast includes eating some protein (preferably lean protein like turkey bacon or sausage), which helps us to feel more satisfied and curbs those sugar cravings. This is known as the "satiation" affect. Not to mention the thermic affect that protein has on the body. In other words, the body burns more calories digesting protein than refined carbo-hydrates (such as cereal), and eating protein helps to reduce muscle tissue loss. Eating eggs for breakfast can also be satisfying, and eggs are actually considered to be a very lean protein.

People that consume large amounts of sugar usually get less of 15 different nutrients than do lighter sugar consumers (under 12 percent of calories) from their diet. The lack of nutrients leads to sugar cravings, and the vicious cycle continues.

Reasons for Sugar Abuse

Keep in mind that eating sweets in moderation is not going to turn you into an "addict." It is simply the abuse of the sweets that can have an addictive affect. And all of the sugar and sweetening food additives and preservatives that a person is not even aware of, can really add to the amount of sweets that the person consumes.

Processed sugars and carbohydrates that turn into sugar cause a rise in the insulin level of the blood, which raises the serotonin level in the brain. (Serotonin improves our mood.) As a result, the sugars cause the person to feel a mental high.

If the person continues to eat large amounts of sugar or carbohydrates, the brain's serotonin sites can slow production of serotonin or close sites in order to regulate the amount of serotonin in the brain. Without the production of serotonin, the person can feel a sense of depression.

So in order to maintain a good mood, the person will eat more sugar and/or carbohydrates to get out of their depression and feel a more normal mood. The effect is similar to the cycle that occurs after excessive dopamine is released into the body from the use of alcohol. Excessive alcohol use causes dopamine sites to shut down, and the alcoholic must drink more alcohol to get the same effect.

The Effect of Low-Fat Diet on Insulin

People who eat a low-fat diet, believing that they will lose weight, can ultimately make the problem worse. Insulin maintains stable blood sugar levels. A low-fat, high carbohydrate diet over a period of time can lead to insulin resistance, which means that the body stops responding to insulin. The result is that the body begins to deposit more calories as fat, making it easier to gain weight.

An insulin resistant person can have continual food cravings, because the cells of the body cannot absorb the glucose that they need since insulin tells the body's cells when to absorb glucose. Insulin resistance results in obesity, diabetes and heart disease.

The effect of sugar on the body does not last long, and usually wears off within an hour. But after the sugar wears off, the effect of insulin is still there. In other words, when eating sugar is stopped, the glut of insulin and the lack of serotonin lead to depression. Along with depression, the body lacks energy. Then the person will eat more sugar in order to feel better.

The lack of energy occurs because the glucose cannot get into the cells for energy, and the cells become "starved." The brain is particularly affected, because the brain's only source of energy is glucose. This starvation causes the brain to signal the body to crave more sugars and carbohydrates.

Also, researchers found that a pattern of overloading on sugary foods sensitizes both dopamine, which creates a feeling of pleasure in rats, and the cycle of deprivation and excessive sugar intake reinforces binging. This is another example of how deprivation does not work.

Dependency on Sugar

According to a study published in Obesity Research, a pattern of fasting and overloading on sugary foods may foster dependence. In addition, those people who have a genetic predisposition for addiction can become overly dependent on sugar.

Eating sweeteners over a period of time can result in a de-sensitization of the taste buds. In other words, our sense of taste becomes so used to the sweet flavor, that whole foods, such as fruits and vegetables, seem bland and tasteless. This also happens with foods that are high in fat, because higher fat foods contain a richer flavor.

The combination of the sweets and the fats really makes us want even more of that rich taste, so we add on more calories. In the end, it becomes difficult to get off of the "treadmill" of constantly eating these types of food. Also, keep in mind that chemical sugar substitutes are not recommended, because they retard the body's ability to lose weight.

Moderation

The good news is that researches have found that withdrawal symptoms and drops in dopamine levels do not exist when meals are moderate and regularly scheduled. Once again, the answer is: Everything in moderation.

Should we never eat cake or other rich foods? Of course not. Deprivation always seems to backfire, and once again we can wind up binging when it comes to those sugary or fattening foods. The Europeans (such as the French women), manage to maintain a healthy weight in spite of eating some of those rich foods, such as a piece of chocolate or cheese. The difference is moderation, and balance.

Achieving Balance

The difference between the foods in America versus other countries, is the amount of processed foods that Americans consume. In other countries, they are enjoying more of the flavors and natural sweetness of whole foods. In other words, foods that have not been processed, but are in their natural state.

It is important to mention that it is really more about the quality of the food, instead of the quantity. Rather than trying to eat a small amount of food, which can slow down the metabolism, try eating more whole foods. In other words, foods that are in their natural form. (An apple is a whole food; a twinkie is not a whole food.) Just walk into your local convenience store, and see if you can find a whole food (with the exception of a few nuts). It's no wonder that Americans have difficulty balancing their weight.

Since sugar is used as an additive and preservative, in order to watch the amount of sugar you eat, simply check the label and choose a similar food that has less sugars. When you check food labels, keep in mind that the larger ingredients are listed first. So if sugar, corn syrup or other sweeteners are near the top of the list, they are probably higher in sugar.

For example, one jar or can of spaghetti sauce may be high in sugar or corn syrup, while another may have none at all. (You are most likely to find the sauce that has no sweeteners at a store that carries more whole or "health" foods.) You may be surprised to find that you enjoy the sauce that has no sweeteners at all, and you will be doing your body (and mind) a favor.

Eating more whole or natural foods may seem tasteless at first, as our taste has actually gotten used to the high-intensity of flavors that are in high-sugar and high-fat foods. The key is patience and stamina (in the beginning). This is because it takes *30 to 90 days* to re-sensitize our sense of taste to where we can enjoy the flavors of foods in their natural form.

Getting through the "withdrawal" of eating those unhealthy foods is well worth the effort. Your taste can then change, and you will begin to crave more natural or whole foods. The rich foods become less appealing, because they actually can taste too "rich" or sweet. As a result, you will not have such a strong desire to eat those foods, and you will look forward to eating more natural foods. The first thing to keep in mind, is that a craving lasts for only 15 seconds. If you can remember that, it can make getting through the initial craving period a little easier.

When alcoholics stop drinking alcohol, they can actually experience a craving for sweets. The amino acid glutamine can help with those cravings. Foods that are rich in glutamine include chicken, beef, fish, beans, eggs and dairy. Also, essential fatty acid supplements that contain omega fatty-acids are important. These fatty-acids come from plants and fish (like salmon), and help to heal the liver and support nerve function.

When people blame themselves for craving sweets or carbohydrates, they simply worsen their mood. The result is an increase in their need for serotonin. Then a pattern of emotional eating can develop. (See the chapter: No pain, no gain.) Not having adequate nutrition can actually result in cravings.

The Right Vitamins and Nutrients to Better Health

Making sure that you are getting enough nutrition, which includes whole foods and quality vitamin and mineral supplements, in addition to moderate exercise, can help curb the cravings. The end result improves the metabolism, without completely giving up those foods that you enjoy. Important nutrients to help curb cravings are:

- ☐ Chromium (contained in broccoli, grapes, cheese, dried beans and chicken).
- ☐ Carbon (found in fresh fruit).
- ☐ Phosphorus (in chicken, beef, liver, poultry, fish, eggs, dairy, nuts, legumes and grains).

☐ Sulphur (contained in cranberries, horseradish, cruciferous vegetables, kale and cabbage).

☐ Tryptophan (cheese, liver, lamb, raisins, sweet potatoes and spinach).

When considering a high-potency multi-vitamin, the following ingredients can help to curb cravings:

☐ Vitamin B1 (Thiamin)
☐ Vitamin B3 (Niacin)
☐ Vitamin B6 (Pyridoxine)
☐ Folic Acid (Folate, Folacin)
☐ Vitamin B12 (Cabalamin, Cyanocoba-lamin, Hydroxocobalamin)
☐ Vitamin C (Ascorbic Acid)
☐ Choline
☐ Magnesium
☐ Calcium

In fact, vitamin deficiency can cause various psychological symptoms (some of which can lead to emotional eating). An iron deficiency anemia (which can especially affect women), can lead to depression and becoming more easily fatigued when exercising. And since exercise can help to balance weight, it is important for women to be able to have enough energy to get the exercise they need.

As mentioned previously, the brain makes its own chemicals to create neurotransmitters like serotonin, in addition to dopamine. These neurotransmitters either start, continue, or stop processes in the brain. It is important to point out the only ingredients that help these processes are vitamins, minerals, fatty acids, amino acids and other nutrients. Without proper nutrition, there can be the wrong combination of neurotransmitters. Some important nutrients are:

1. **Essential Fatty Acids** — This nutrient is essential to the healthy creation of structures such as cell membranes. They are necessary for brain development in addition to nerve transmission. A deficiency of this nutrient can be bipolar disorder, depression, aggression and general mental function.

2. **Vitamin B6** — This vitamin helps to form neurotransmitters. The deficiency of vitamin B6 can be depression, irritability, agitation and general impairment of mental function.

3. **Zinc** — It is believed to be a neurotransmitter, and a deficiency in Zinc can cause feelings of anger, memory problems,

immunity impairment, decreased mental function, and difficulty dealing with stress.

For many people, eating sugar can give them the "sugar blues."(Sugar actually uses many important nutrients when the body processes it.) To get the correct nutrient balance, it is recommended that you talk to a professional, such as a naturopathic medical doctor who can recommend nutrients that your body may need. Testing may determine that a person's body does not absorb nutrition well, or there may be various other factors that can lead to a lack of adequate nutrition.

The Effect of Stress

The sweets "cycle"is also affected by stress. When the body is under stress, the stress hormone called cortisol is produced. Cortisol increases insulin production, which gives the person the same feeling as eating too much sugar or carbohydrates. In fact, a Georgetown University study revealed that stress chemicals in the brain cause the same reaction as in drug addiction, that makes people want pleasurable things in excess.

It was found that when rats were given cues for the same treats the stress chemical in the brain increased the intense desire for sugary foods by three times the normal desire. In other words, when the rats had a similar level of stress chemicals in their brain that humans have when they are stressed, they had a higher craving for a sugar reward. The stress chemicals can make people feel a greater feeling of temptation, making them want to consume sugary foods that they normally could resist. (For stress reduction tips, see the chapter called: Breathe.)

Safe Alternative Sweeteners

There are other sweeteners that are available (besides the common artificial sweeteners) that are more natural and are better for you. One of those sweeteners is Stevia and another is Xylitol, which is a naturally occurring sweetener that is found in the fibers of many fruits and vegetables such as oats, corn husks, berries and mushrooms. It can be extracted from birch trees, plums, raspberries and corn. Actually, our bodies produce up to 15 grams of xylitol in a day by metabolizing various foods. Xylitol has only two-thirds the food energy of sucrose, but has about the same sweetness.

Xylitol was originally extracted from birch trees in Finland in the 19thcentury, and has been used in Europe as a safe alternative sweetener for diabetics. It is safe for people with diabetes and hyperglycemia because it is a sugar alcohol, which does not have the effect that sugar does on blood sugar levels, and it is absorbed more slowly than sugar. A teaspoon of Xylitol has 9.6 calories, compared to sugar which has 15 calories. Also, Xylitol has no net effective carbohydrates, unlike sugar which has four grams per five ml.

Xylitol can be found in some chewing gums and breath mints, because it does not promote tooth decay. It also has a plaque-reducing effect because it attracts and then starves micro-organisms in the mouth, so that the mouth can re-mineralize damaged teeth. Researchers have discovered that xylitol helps to prevent weakening bones, and improves bone density, which is good news for the prevention of osteoporosis.

Other health benefits of xylitol includes its ability to help control oral infections of Candida yeast, and the prevention of ear infections as it prevents the growth of bacteria in the Eustachian tubes which connect the nose and the ear. (It is available as a saline nasal wash that contains xylitol.) If xylitol is consumed in large amounts, it can have a laxative effect like most sugar alcohols because it is not fully broken down when it is digested. There are no known toxic levels of xylitol when it comes to human consumption. However, it is important to keep xylitol away from dogs, as it can be toxic to them.

Like organic food, xylitol costs more than sugar, but the health benefits are worth the price.

Balance by Choice

Ultimately our cravings affect what we put in our body, and what we put in our body (or what we don't put in our body in the case of not enough nutrients) can create more cravings. The result is a vicious cycle of consuming large amounts of sweets and other rich foods that fuel our cravings, which negatively affects our weight, not to mention how we feel mentally and emotionally.

We have a choice: We can simply pay more attention to what "added"ingredients are in our food, in addition to adding some nutrients along with eating more natural foods the way nature intended. We can feel better mentally and physically. Then, both our cravings and our weight can become balanced. Having that balance allows us to re-connect with ourselves, so that we can find our own natural feeling of joy instead of the artificial highs and lows that are created by our out-of-control cravings.

4

Love: The Main Ingredient

One word frees us of all the weight and pain of life:
That word is love.
— Sophocles (496 BC – 406 BC)

*L*ike the Beatles said, "all you need is love."
When it comes to food, we could certainly use a
little. Back when life wasn't so hectic, our
ancestors were known to put a little love in the
food that they prepared. When grandma
sprinkled in her spices, she also added some
love. And that love went a long way.

Food Preparation

Today, people have a tendency to prepare foods
quickly. Everything is fast, including fixing our
food. As a result, the preparation of meals often
becomes mechanical, and lacking in the positive
energy and taste that people before us added to

their meals. And of course, we know how the fast food chains throw their food together. That is food that is *empty of love*, and contains *empty calories*. The love and appreciation that should go into preparing food has become a thing of the past for many people today.

Do you think that processed foods contain much love? These foods are generally created by machine. They lack the main ingredients necessary to provide you with calories that are full, rather than empty. Food is prepared mechanically for those on the go. It may be convenient to just fill the stomach without nourishing the body. People who are working as fast as they can are the ones who prepare the food, and what mood are they in at that time? If a cook puts more time and attention into the food, it will contain more positive energy. It stands to reason that food being nurtured as it is prepared will be more nurturing to our bodies and our souls. Maybe that's why they call it: Soul Food.

The Food Connection

After all, food is not simply a commodity, but a way that we connect with the earth. It helps to define who we are through our community and our culture. It is part of our holiday celebrations, and helps us to connect with each other and nature. Today, many people are going back to "whole foods" knowing that is a more healthy way of eating, and it helps to reconnect with the earth.

We are energy. So think of love as energy. Everything around us has energy in it. Chi or positive energy is the vital force that sustains us and animates us. We get most of our chi energy through the air that we breathe, but food is the second most important way in which energy is taken into the body.

Fresh foods carry a life force, which has been seen through Kirlian photography. Fresh fruits and vegetables that were photographed soon after they were picked have a glow around them. Processed foods have a depleted charge, or no Chi energy at all. The way that food is grown, stored and cooked will affect the life-force-energy of the food.

The Energy of Plants

Plants not only provide us with life-sustaining food, they provide us with a life-force energy. They can brighten a room, and provide oxygen in a sterile environment. And when they are nurtured, they respond to our love and care. This nurturing is something that gardeners find to be very therapeutic, so that the love and care not only goes to the plants, but also to the humans who take care of them. That can be healing for both mind and body.

Emotions and the Way we Eat

What we eat and how we prepare it can have an effect on our emotions. That energy (which can be positive or negative) can be transferred through what we eat. For example, it has actually been determined that there is a biochemical aspect to anger. The roots of anger are in our body and also in our mind. The body and mind are not separate — the mind is the body. Therefore, what happens to the body also happens to the mind. As a result, the physical and mental aspect of anger is not separate.

The way we grow our food, the way we eat and what we put in our bodies can have a profound effect on how we feel. For example, in the old days, chickens roamed free on people's farms, pecking away at the food they were given. In today's society, chickens are raised on large farms in cages where they cannot walk, or find their food on the ground as they once did. They have to stand at all times. How would you feel if you had to stand in one place all of the time?

Artificial days and nights are created to produce more eggs with indoor lighting, and the chickens never see the true light of day.

Because of this, it can be said that the chickens are frustrated or even angry. They express their anger by pecking the chickens that are next to them — pecking with their beaks and wounding each other. Farms end up cutting part of the beaks off of the chickens to prevent them from hurting each other.

The question then becomes: Can this anger be passed into your body when you eat it? It is believed that happy eggs come from happy chickens. Some people choose to eat chicken and eggs that are from "cage free"or "free range"chickens. Certain animals, such as goats, only thrive when they are free to roam.

Overeating can cause problems for the digestive system, which can contribute to the physical, and ultimately the mental anger that we may feel. Too much eating can cause too much energy, and this excessive energy can result in anger. And it is believed that depression is anger "turned inward."

The Benefit of Natural Organic Food

Organic milk comes from cows that are raised naturally, and in a humane way. Cows that are grass fed instead of fed with pesticide-sprayed grains produce raw organic dairy products that have natural anti-inflammatory nutrients in them. This is because of the fat that is contained in those natural organic products. (Eating food that has anti-inflammatory nutrients could help ease the symptoms of arthritis.) Also, the cows that are producing organic milk are not fed hormones, to fatten them up.

Some people have discovered that even though they are lactose intolerant and are unable to eat dairy products, *are* able to drink raw organic milk that has not been pasteurized. Those people may find that raw milk gives them more energy, and improves their mood, even to the point of alleviating symptoms of depression. For some, only eating organic foods can help with their feelings of anxiety and depression. This is because some people are sensitive to pesticides and other food additives.

Mass-produced food such as fruits and vegetables are sometimes grown in devitalized soil, and can lack the nutrients of home-grown fruits and vegetables tended with love and care. Purchasing organic produce can help us to get more of those nutrients that people used to get from their lovingly home-grown food. It may cost more, but we can appreciate it more, and perhaps enjoy eating it more (and more sparingly). Eating smaller amounts of high quality organic foods and supporting the farmers that raise the healthy food that we eat (whether it is meat or produce) is a more natural way to be good to our bodies and our minds.

How Human Energy can Affect Water

Masaru Emoto is a Japanese researcher who has been studying messages from water for several years, and what those messages are trying to tell us. His research involves the impact that thoughts have on the formation of water crystals. He has discovered that human vibrational energy, thoughts, words, ideas and music, affect the molecular structure of water. (Our bodies are comprised of over 70 percent water, and about the same percentage of water covers the planet.) Water is the source of all life on the planet.

The energy or vibrations from the environment can change the molecular shape of water. Its physical appearance changes, and the molecular shape also changes. Mr. Emoto has documented the molecular changes using photographs. Droplets of water are frozen, and then examined under a microscope that has photographic capabilities.

Mr. Emoto has discovered many fascinating differences in the crystalline structures of water from may different sources and conditions around the planet. Fresh water from mountain streams have beautifully formed geometric designs in their crystalline patterns. Polluted and toxic water from industrial and populated areas have distorted and randomly formed crystalline structures.

Mr. Emoto studied the effects that different types of music has on the formation of crystals. He then decided to see how thoughts and words affected the formation of untreated distilled water crystals, using words typed onto paper by a word processor and taped on glass bottles overnight. The water molecules from negative words were distorted, indicating that water responds to thoughts and emotions.

It became clear that water easily takes on the vibrations and energy of its environment. And, since most of our food contains water (as we do), we can consider the effect that the transference of negative energy to our food can have on our bodies.

Electricity and its Effect on Food

It has been said that using electricity can change the energy of food. The intense vibration of microwave ovens can also affect the cellular integrity of our food, thereby we absorb the negative result when we eat it. Medical studies show that microwaved food can produce major changes in blood and immune function.

Energetically, it can contribute to the damage, deterioration and decomposition of body cells. Electric cooking is not as powerful as microwave cooking, but it is believed that major changes in energy can lead to erratic digestive, circulatory and nervous functions. It can produce an overall weakening effect, which can include a loss of mental focus and concentration. Once again, quickly prepared food may not be such a good thing.

Natural and Organic Food

Mother Nature naturally puts a lot of love, or positive energy in her food. Natural, and especially organic food is higher in vitamins and fiber, which is healthier for our bodies. As Edgar Cayce said: "Eat the foods that carry these vitamins, rather than adding the vitamins."

The more processed that food becomes, the less healthy it is, as it is taken further away from nature. The more that it is mashed, strained, cooked, sugared and filled with corn syrup, the more fattening it becomes. As the natural vitamins and fiber are taken out, the less healthy it becomes. This is why whole foods are so important. If we can eat the way that nature intended, we would receive the nutrition and loving ingredients that our bodies deserve.

The positive energy that is contained in our food, also depends on the way we prepare it and the way we cook it. And, eating relates to the flow of energy, and is a way that we receive energy. This is why the way that we handle food should be done in a loving way.

When we wash our food, we can provide some positive energy by feeling the love of caring for the food that we will be eating. That positive intention can then flow into the food that we put into our bodies. Instead of worrying and feeling stressed, just take a moment to breathe and enjoy the process of cleansing the food with the water, and with positive feelings.

Those feelings will be transferred into the tasty home-cooked meal that we create. After all, thoughts are truly part of us, and positive emotions help to fill those empty calories, allowing us to feel more satisfied.

In other words, be fully present when you are preparing your food, just like you should be when you are eating. Enjoy the moment. Be in the "now." Take a deep breath, and relax as you prepare and cook your food. Use that time to de-stress. Being mindful of the moment can go along way in satisfying our appetite for food and for life.

When it comes to lovingly preparing beverages, consider the Trappestine monks of Belgium. Those monks pour a lot of heart and soul into the brewing of their beer, as they take the time to lovingly create it. As a result, it is known to be some of the best tasting beer in the world.

Cooking with Happy Memories

Cooking itself can be very creative, and can be a time to reflect and remember good times. Do you have fond memories of cooking with a relative? Perhaps your mother, father, grandmother, or anyone else that you have been close to? Or perhaps you remember the smell of that good home-cooked food when you were growing up. We can often recall the fond memories of a nice holiday meal and a favorite family recipe.

Why not take out one of those classic family recipes, and enjoy the moment of cooking with the positive memory of someone that you love. You can share that time with your children, and talk about the positive memories that you have from the time you were younger. Or, you can share those positive thoughts with anyone else in your life that you enjoy spending time with.

These memories help us to re-connect with those we love. It brings us closer to our sense of self. It allows us to remember who we are and where we came from, and that connection that we had with our mother, or another family member.

If those memories are not positive for you, then why not create some new memories about food? Find or create some classic recipes for yourself and your loved ones. Make cooking and meals a time to connect with those people that you love. And if you are eating alone, it can be a time to simply relax, take a deep breath, and enjoy the time with yourself, enjoying the nourishment that each tasty bite provides to your mind, body and soul.

Energy Balanced Foods

The Asian art of feng shui is all about harmony and energy-balanced food. That balance includes variety and a balance of colors. A yin and yang balanced dish would contain strong flavors as well as delicate flavors. Yin foods include sweeteners, oil liquids, and most dairy products. These foods have a cooling and lethargic effect on people.

Some foods provide an initial burst of energy. However, this energy can become a letdown. Caffeine, alcohol, and various drugs are in this group. Yang foods include meat, salt, eggs and hard cheeses, which have a heating and animating effect on the body. Too much of these foods results in tension and rigidity. You need balance.

It is common in the western culture to consume large amounts of either yin or yang food, which results in an imbalance in the body's energy that ultimately manifests into physical problems. This is another reason why diets that include eating larger amounts of a certain type of food, or excluding entire categories of food, creates an imbalance in the body. Ultimately, once again, our bodies will want that balance, as we crave the foods that we are lacking.

Feng shui also teaches that you should like the smell of your food. Every sense including flavors, colors and smells should balance. Every sense that is part of the eating process should be paid attention to. Chinese physicians believe that food is a constant cure. First, they try food, and *then* resort to medication, only when food fails to effect a cure. And a lovingly prepared, home-cooked meal can be just what the doctor ordered.

Benefits of Cooking Ahead

Although it may seem as though there is not enough time, if we can somehow take a few moments to add that love into our meals, we can once again enjoy the love and care that our bodies deserve. This nourishment can then nurture our bodies the way they should be nurtured, positively affecting our mind, and connecting us to our sense of self.

You may be thinking: "I don't have time to cook fresh meals every night!"In that case, consider cooking larger quantities of good homemade recipes on the weekend, and then freezing them in separate containers. (Some people call it "make ahead meals.") If you do this once per week, over time you can accumulate a variety of homemade frozen foods that are made from scratch, and not processed. This can also be done once per month, where you can cook several recipes and freeze them.

The dinners can be taken out of the freezer the night before, so they are thawed for the next day. They can also be put in individual size containers for lunch. Microwaving food may be unavoidable, especially at work. However at home, the food can be heated in a pan or a toaster oven. Cooking in larger quantities is not only easier on your body, it's also easier on your pocketbook. (Especially when you have children to feed.) It allows you to buy in bulk, which can be cheaper by the pound. For example, meat can cost less by the pound when it is purchased in larger quantities. It also saves time in the long run, by cutting down on meal preparation each day.

Another way to prepare meals for the freezer is to double the meal size each night for a week, and you will have another seven meals in your freezer. You can keep doing this as long as you can, and continue to create home prepared meals that can be frozen.

Before you know it, you will have enough meals so that you will not have to cook for awhile. (Many recipes for bulk cooking can be found on the Internet by using search words such as: Once a month cooking, or once a week cooking.) You will soon find that you are enjoying those lovingly prepared home-cooked meals. You may find that you are eating healthier, and in less quantities than before, since fast food or restaurant meals can be larger, and the ingredients can certainly be less healthy.

The way that we should eat all goes back to balance and moderation. So, enjoy the foods that you love in moderation, and prepare them with some positive energy. Try to eat some wholesome food that is as close to nature as possible. Savor the variety of tastes, textures, and smells. Love your food, and it will love and nurture you.

5

Breathe

Breathe. Let go. And remind yourself that this very moment is the only one you know you have for sure.

– Oprah Winfrey

Stress is Harmful

Today's stress-prone lifestyle has had an impact on the continuing weight issues that society has been experiencing. Stress can affect a person's emotional balance, which can lead to weight imbalance. It can take away the ability to think clearly, function properly, and enjoy life. Ultimately the connection among the various issues, including stress and obesity, has led to a disconnection with ourselves.

The body reacts to stress when any change that requires an adjustment or response occurs. The reactions by the body include physical, mental and emotional responses. Although stress is a normal part of life, too much stress can cause our bodies to react in unhealthy ways. Keep in mind that stress can occur even from positive changes, such as getting married. But too much stress without taking time for relief and relaxation can lead to stress-related problems.

Common acute stressors include noise, crowding, isolation, hunger, danger, infection, imagining a threat or remembering a dangerous event. When the threat has passed, the levels of stress hormones return to normal. This is called the relaxation response. However, when stressful situations last too long, then stress becomes chronic. The most common chronic stressors are: pressures at work, on-going relationship problems, loneliness and continued financial worries.

It is an interesting fact that after the 9/11 terrorist attacks, 15 percent of Americans were turning to comfort food, and 14 percent of the population indicated that they were eating more sweets. Ten percent of Americans had gained weight within two months of the terrorist attacks.

The normal ups and downs that we experience in our modern day lives can lead to the use of food to try to relieve the symptoms of stress, including anxiety and depression. Certain foods can help us feel better, such as sweets and fats. Stored fat sends out a metabolic signal that goes to the brain, which tells the brain to shut off the stress response. As a result, the symptoms of stress are reduced (at least temporarily).

These high-calorie foods that we may be self-medicating with seem to make us feel better temporarily, but they are not good for our long-term health. In ancient times, our fight-or-flight response to stress made us run, which was much better for our health than eating comfort foods. Instead, we wind up storing more fat rather than burning the fat that we already have. Once again, we have lost the connection with who we are, and how our bodies were designed.

Stress can lead to sleep disturbances like insomnia. The resulting fatigue can slow down the metabolism, which can make it harder for a person to get their weight in balance. And when a person is tired, they are less likely to get the exercise they need to help burn excess fat from those stress-relieving comfort foods.

Chronic stress can even cause weight gain in people who are eating a balanced diet. In some people who are feeling stressed, the weight that is gained is often abdominal fat, which is the kind that leads to diabetes and heart problems. It is the release of the stress hormone cortisol that appears to promote abdominal fat. Besides weight gain, eating disorders such as anorexia nervosa and bulimia can be related to adjustment problems in response to stress and emotional issues.

The following are some tips for coping with stress related eating:

1. **Eat regularly, including breakfast.** Hunger is an acute stressor, and eating some breakfast can put you in a better mood.

2. **Evaluate your hunger.** Are you actually hungry, or are you really stressed? Recognize your stress signals, which could be a headache, a change in breathing, or some other physical symptom.

3. **Do not wait until you are starving.** Break your food down to several smaller meals rather than one or two large meals. Eating a large meal can deprive the brain of oxygen that is needed for digestion, which can make you feel tired.

4. **Learn from your experiences.** Did you feel guilty the last time you over-indulged? As you are reminded of this, try controlling the portion by eating one instead of several of that treat that you are thinking of eating.

5. **Write down what you eat**. When people eat out of stress, they may not be aware of the food that they ate.

6. **Don't ignore your cravings.** A craving lasts for about 15 seconds. So, you can try to give yourself a little time, and you may find that you will become occupied with something other than food. However, if the craving returns, and you continue to deny the craving, simply acknowledge the craving and give yourself a choice. Do you want to satisfy the craving with a little something now, or wait until you end up inhaling too much of that treat later? If you give yourself a choice, it puts you in charge.

7. **Stop stressing about food.** If you really feel the need, then have a snack, and then let go of any stressful feelings.

8. **Try putting a post-it note in places where you may get stressed,** such as in your car, on your computer or mirror, or any place that

may be a good reminder to ask yourself: "Am I really hungry?"

9. **Exercise.** Take a walk, hop on a treadmill, or exercise bike, or go outside and ride a bike. Get some form of exercise which might include a sport that you enjoy.

10. **Reduce caffeine and sugar.** These two ingredients cause a temporary "high," which result in a crash in mood and energy. This can lead to more cravings.

However, if we simply stop the stress eating without dealing with the cause of the stress, it can create other physical issues such as putting added strain on the heart. This is because the emotional stress makes the heart work harder. For those people who have heart related problems, it is especially important for them to release their stress.

Consider that 43 percent of adults suffer from adverse health effects from stress. 75 to 90 percent of the complaints with doctor's visits are stress related. In addition to obesity and heart problems, stress can cause headaches, high blood pressure, diabetes, asthma, arthritis, anxiety and depression. The costs of stress on corporate America is more than $300 billion annually.

Sometimes people are dealing with constant stress, especially if they are a "Type A" personality, which is someone who is a perfectionist, or someone who is constantly worrying or juggling too many demands. Sometimes they feel they are reaching the breaking point. And people can be stressed from a variety of issues such as rush hour traffic, their job, family issues or finances. This does not only affect a person's health, but their peace of mind.

Stress management involves identifying the sources of stress in your life. Keep in mind that the source of the stress may not always be obvious. Sometimes the cause of the stress can be your own thoughts, feelings and behaviors. For example, it may be your procrastination rather than the job deadlines that ultimately creates the stress.

In addition to eating high-fat or sugary foods, people sometimes have other unhealthy ways of dealing with stress such as: Smoking, self-medicating with alcohol or drugs, using prescription tranquilizers, sleeping too much, procrastination, or withdrawing from family, friends or activities.

The physical warning signs of too much stress include: Feeling dizzy or feeing "out of it,"experiencing various aches and pains, clenching your jaw or grinding your teeth, headaches, indigestion, a change in appetite, muscle tension in the shoulders, neck or back, insomnia, a racing heart, sweaty or cold hands, exhaustion, trembling or shaking, upset stomach, or unexpected weight gain or loss.

Stress Management

It is important to keep in mind that there will always be bills, and there will always be twenty-four hours in a day. If you are stressed, then simply realizing that you are in control of your life can be the beginning of managing your stress. Either way, managing stress requires change. You can either change the situation, or change your reaction to the situation. You can start by asking yourself what makes you feel calm and in control.

Coping strategies for dealing with stress in general include:

1. **Connecting with others.** Get some support by talking to family, friends or clergy. And/or join a support group.

2. **Adjust your standards.** If you demand perfection, then you may be setting yourself up for failure. Set reasonable standards for yourself and others.

3. **Get enough sleep.** If you are tired, it can increase your stress because it may cause you to think irrationally.

4. **Express your feelings.** Communicate in a respectful way to avoid having pent-up anger.

5. **If you feel anger**, take a deep breath and give yourself a moment to calm down.

6. **Set aside some time for yourself to relax.** Include doing something that you enjoy every day.

7. **Take control of your environment.** If you get stressed from the evening news, then turn it off. If going shopping stresses you, then try shopping online.

8. **Keep a journal about what causes your stress**, how you felt when you were stressed, how you reacted, and what you can do to cope with or what you can do to change the situation.

9. **Try some meditation to increase your awareness.** (See the meditation tips in this chapter.)

10. **Remember the serenity prayer:** God grant me the serenity to accept the things I cannot

change, the courage to change the things I can, and the wisdom to know the difference.

11. **Practice appreciation**, by focusing on the positive aspects of life. (Each day, write down at least three things that you are appreciative of in your journal.)

12. **Try to avoid situations that you know will stress you**, such as changing your schedule to avoid rush hour traffic.

13. **Learn to say "no."** If you feel that you are being "spread too thin," then you may want to put a limit on what you are willing to do. In addition to taking care of others, it is also important to take care of yourself.

If you are unable to get help from any of these suggestions, you may benefit by getting help from a professional counselor. Your family, friends, or doctor may be able to recommend someone who can help you to sort out your stress issues.

The Importance of Laughter

Another way to relieve stress is through laughter, which reduces cortisol (a hormone that causes stress, and can also elevate blood sugar levels). Laughter increases endorphins, which make a person feel happy. To also combat stress, laughter secretes an enzyme that protects the stomach from forming ulcers. Besides relieving stress, laughing ten to fifteen minutes a day can burn an extra 40 calories. Other benefits of laughter include: Anti-aging by reducing the rate of cellular decay, improving mental function, alertness, memory and interpersonal responsiveness.

Laughter improves immunity, by increasing the body's T-cell count. (T-cells are a type of white blood cell and are part of the immune system. They kill outside invading bacteria that are harmful to the body.) During flu season, consider that laughing can increase antibodies in saliva, which combat upper respiratory infections.

Laugher helps blood vessels to function better, it reduces blood pressure and heart rate, aids ventilation, enhances blood oxygen levels (which can help to burn fat) and boosts circulation. And, laughter can be considered an exercise, since it conditions the abdominal muscles. It can also help to relax the muscles throughout the body, relieving stress-related tension.

Norman Cousins was an author, journalist, professor and an advocate for world peace who lived from 1912-1990. During his life he received nearly 50 honorary degrees and numerous awards. He researched the biochemistry of human emotions, and believed that positive emotion allowed people to overcome illnesses. He lived for many years with heart disease, and in 1977 he contracted cancer. Eventually his cancer went into remission, as he used his "laugh-cure" along with love, faith, hope and a positive attitude.

Watching Marx Brothers films, Norman said "I made the joyous discovery that ten minutes of genuine belly laughter had an anesthetic affect and would give me at least two hours of pain-free sleep." He also saw laughter as exercise, stating that "hearty laughter is a good way to jog internally without having to go outdoors."

Physical Activities

One of the most important aspects of stress management is to work it out with physical activity. If you can "let loose" with exercise, it will give you stronger bones and muscles, increase your metabolism, give you more energy and help you to resist illness. In the case of stress, you can let off some steam. It distracts you from the source of the stress, and it improves your mood.

People who get regular physical activity generally eat better. Eating better helps to manage the stress, and you will most likely lose weight in the process. Competition can really help to get rid of pent-up stress hormones. Try asking a friend if they would like to play some tennis, racquetball or try some other sport. Dancing is a great enjoyable way of exercise — you could join a dance club.

An exercise "buddy" can help to provide the motivation you need if you don't feel like you have the energy to exercise. Just remember to set realistic goals. Physical activity can certainly reduce stress, but overdoing it can make it worse. Don't let the idea of having to work out "stress you out." Above all, the question is: What would you enjoy doing? Because getting some exercise should be enjoyable and energizing. (See the chapter on fitness for mind, body and soul.)

If you work with a lot of people and prefer to exercise alone, you might try a home video. (Keep in mind that it is always good to check with your doctor, especially if you have certain physical issues that need to be considered.) Next thing you know, your worries will be left behind, along with a couple of pounds of stored energy (fat).

Foods that Can Relieve Stress

Other ways of reducing stress and its negative effect on weight management, is to try some foods or beverages that have stress-relieving benefits. The following foods can help ease the tension and stress that you may be feeling:

Tea: There are certain teas that can be relaxing. Researchers have found that people who drink black tea are able to let go of their stress more quickly than people who drank a tea substitute. The reason that black tea works is because it contains certain ingredients that reduce levels of the stress hormone cortisol. Also, Chamomile tea helps to relax nerves. (It also boosts immunity to help relieve cold symptoms and can reduce menstrual cramps.)

Nuts: Try snacking on a few nuts to reduce stress. Nuts are high in tryptophan and magnesium, which produce serotonin (a neurotransmitter that helps with relaxation, sleep and concentration).

Vitamin C: Eating foods that are high in vitamin C can also reduce stress. Besides citrus fruits like oranges, try some kiwi fruit. Other foods that contain vitamin C are tomatoes, potatoes, and broccoli. Also, try spicing things up with some yellow, orange or red peppers, which also contain vitamin C.

Berries: Tasty berries contain powerful antioxidants and also have vitamin C. The antioxidants help to neutralize free radicals, which are highly unstable oxygen molecules that can damage normal cells. (Try some blueberries or blackberries).

Complex carbs: Whole grain foods are not only great for fiber, but they also boost serotonin levels and help to keep you feeling calm and relaxed. Try some oatmeal, brown rice, whole grain breads, and legumes such as peas, beans and lentils.

B Vitamins: During times of stress, B vitamins help maintain regular blood sugar levels. They support the immune system, the adrenal glands and the entire nervous system. Foods that contain B vitamins include eggs, fresh meats, unprocessed grains, salmon, nuts, corn, soy, citrus fruit, lentils and sunflower seeds.

Try spreading your eating evenly through-out the day. By eating several smaller, lighter meals, you will keep your metabolism going while feeling more alert than if you ate one or two large meals. Start with breakfast, a mid-morning snack, a light lunch, a mid-afternoon snack (possibly fruit) and a moderate dinner. An evening snack is also OK. Again, depriving or "starving" yourself is not the answer.

Sometimes the process of cooking can actually help to relieve stress, and can take the place of excessive eating. But instead of cooking baked goods, you can try making a soup or a classic family recipe, which can help to feed the mind, and the soul. (See the chapter called Love: The Main Ingredient.) If you cook something that takes some time to prepare, that enjoyment of putting it together can take the place of eating. Also, remember to make sure you are getting enough vitamins.

Aromatherapy, Breathing and Meditation

Another way of de-stressing is to use some aromatherapy. There are a variety of relaxing scents that can be used to help you to feel more relaxed. Calming scents include: vanilla, lavender, lemon balm and chamomile. Also, taking the time for a massage or a facial can be very relaxing in times of tension and stress.

It is a known fact that learning how to breathe correctly can relieve stress. And since the word aerobic refers to getting air or oxygen, then aerobic exercise provides oxygen to the body, which is also important for calorie burning. If a person is unable to get much exercise due to physical limitations, they might consider a breathing meditation. And, it has been discov-ered that meditating is actually effective for anyone who is trying to achieve and maintain a healthy weight.

A Swiss study discovered that people given nutrition education and guidance along with training in meditation lost on average twice as much weight as those given only nutrition and diet guidance. Another study by Dr. Jean Kristeller used meditation-based eating aware-ness therapy (MB-EAT) to treat obesity. She found that people who never thought they would be able to permanently change their eating habits actually transformed their rela-tionships with food. While a person achieves a healthy weight with the help of meditation, they also receive many other mental and physical benefits.

The calming affects of meditation can alter biochemical functions, and lower the body's oxygen demand, blood lactic acid level, carbon dioxide production, heart and respiration rates and blood fatty acid levels. Neuroscientists have found that people who meditate are able to shift their brain activity from the stress-prone right frontal section to the more calm left frontal area of the brain. This shift can decrease the effects of stress, mild depression and anxiety. There can also be less activity in the part of the mind that processes fear. In fact, it has been discovered that people who meditated were generally calmer, and felt happier after eight weeks of mediation.

Also, meditation can improve concentration. Even professional athletes use meditation, since the increased ability to concentrate can improve their performance level in sports. (The improved performance may motivate a person to continue with a particular sport, which can improve their level of fitness, and help to balance their weight.) Meditation also increases a heart patient's ability to exercise.

Meditation can reduce anxiety attacks, lower muscle tension, reduce headaches, increase serotonin production for a better mood, and it can help with chronic diseases such as allergies and arthritis. In addition, Meditation helps to deal with pre-menstrual syndrome, helps patients to heal after an operation, improves the immune system to lower the activity of viruses, and it increases the activity of cells that kill bacteria and cancer cells.

When we think and analyze, we can get caught up in focusing on the past or the future. This continual thinking can take away our sense of creativity and spontaneity. By quieting the mind through meditation, we can clear a path to creativity. It brings us into the "now." In doing so, we can tap into our true potential. This is evident when you consider the great thinkers and scientists who made important discoveries during their creating process by not being interrupted by other thoughts.

Meditation can help us to fill the emptiness inside, which can be the cause of a person's emotional eating. But to be successful at it, it is important to be persistent. It takes time to learn to quiet the mind, and to achieve all of these benefits. But if the quietness is achieved, a purer form of inner peace can be discovered. The end result is that the person will eventually be able to stay happy all the time, even in some of the most difficult circumstances. Some people call this state "nirvana."

Proper meditation requires a comfortable cushion, and a good posture. The posture includes keeping your back straight. This can be achieved by having a cushion where the back part of it is higher than the front, which inclines the pelvis slightly forward. Although it is not necessary to sit cross-legged, it is a good idea to sit this way if you can do it comfortably. If not, then try to sit in a position that is as close to cross-legged as possible.

Next, you can place your right hand in the left hand, with the palms facing up and the thumbs slightly raised and touching. The hands can be held about four fingers' width below the navel. This helps you to concentrate. The back should be straight, but not tense, so that you can develop and maintain a clear mind. Keeping your mouth closed, the tongue should touch the back of the upper teeth. (This prevents excessive salivation, and also prevents your mouth from becoming too dry.)

Your head can be tipped a little forward with the chin slightly tucked in, with your eyes looking down. Your eyes should not be either wide open, or completely closed. Instead, they should be half open, and should gaze down in the same direction as your nose. Keeping the eyes open can be distracting, and completely closing them may cause you to go too deep. Your shoulders should be level, and your elbows can be held slightly away from your body in order to keep air circulating.

After you become comfortable in your meditation position, you should start to become aware of thoughts that are coming up in your mind. When that happens, think instead about your breathing, while you continue to breathe normally. When you exhale, imagine that you are releasing any disturbing thoughts in the form of black smoke, which disappears as it drifts away from you.

When you breathe in, imagine that you are breathing in a feeling of inspiration in the form of white light that goes into your lungs and to your heart. You can continue to visualize this inhaling of white light and exhaling of black smoke twenty-one times, or until your mind has become peaceful and alert. Because you are focused on your breathing, negative thoughts will temporarily disappear. This is because the mind cannot concentrate on more than one thought at a time. The end result will be a sense of calm and a feeling of de-stressing. Your mind is also clearer for you to imagine more positive thoughts that can inspire you, rather than distress you.

Some people simply use numbered breathing to reduce stress. You can do this by slowly inhaling for seven seconds, and slowly exhaling for eight seconds. (Try rocking from heel to toe as you breathe.) When you are counting as you breathe, it brings you into the present and eliminates stressful thoughts by making you focus on the numbers.

To take action in managing your stress, you can set your stress-management goals. You can start by writing an action plan in your journal. Try the following steps:

1. Write down a list of things that cause you to stress.

2. Write down one that you know you can change. (Example: Get more sleep.)

3. Then write a goal for that stressor, such as: I will go to bed a half hour earlier, and write down what time that will be.

4. You can also create a timeframe to reach that goal, which could be: Starting on Monday I will go to bed at: (whatever time you have chosen).

Once again, it can take three weeks to make or break a habit that was previously created, so remember to be patient with yourself. You may want to focus on a smaller goal first, so that you can achieve it. You can also keep notes on your progress by writing them down in your journal. A stress-management buddy can also help. When you have created a healthy new habit for reducing stress, it can be helpful to reward yourself. Think of a mini-vacation, or something simple like a massage that can actually reduce your stress even more.

You can also write an affirmation, which can be one sentence that includes that goal. That affirmation should always be in the present tense, so your mind does not think of it as being in the future but being in the now. It could be: I am reducing my stress by going to bed at 9:00 p.m., which allows me to feel more relaxed and rested.

You can also program yourself to sleep more deeply. The affirmation could be: I am getting plenty of rest, and when I wake up in the morning, I feel refreshed and energized. When you create an affirmation, you can put it on a post-it note and place the note where you will see it most often. You might want to put it near your bed, and read it at bedtime, so that your subconscious mind will remember it, as you drift off to sleep.

Keep in mind, that the right answer for reducing stress, is the one that works for you. Whatever *feels* right to you, is the correct solution to your situation. And by reducing the stress, you can manage your weight more effectively, without creating more tension with diets that do not work for you.

And finally, the Ten Commandments for stress reduction are:

I. Thou shalt not be perfect, or even try to be.

II. Thou shalt not try to be all things to all people.

III. Thou shalt sometimes leave things undone.

IV. Thou shalt not spread thyself too thin.

V. Thou shalt learn to say "no."

VI. Thou shalt schedule time for thyself.

VII. Thou shalt relax, and do nothing regularly.

VIII. Thou shalt not even feel guilty for doing nothing, or saying no.

IX. Thou shalt find support in others.

X. Especially, thou shalt love thyself and be thine own best friend.

6

Fitness for Mind, Body and Soul

Why do strong arms fatigue themselves with frivolous dumbbells? To dig a vineyard is worthier exercise for men.
– Marcus Valerius Martialis (40 AD – 103 AD)

If you think of your body as if it were your car, you can imagine that the fuel that is kept in the tank is like the fat that is stored in your fat cells (which are like tiny fuel tanks). After all, fat is stored energy, and your muscles are like the engine in your car. The simplest way to use that stored energy is to get the muscles going. In other words, get in your "car" and take it for a nice drive.

We know that it is not good to let a car sit for a long period of time, as the fuel lines can clog up, and the car gets to the point where it no longer runs. Dieting slows the metabolism, which is kind of what happens when you let a vehicle sit around without being used. In a similar way, our metabolism can slow down to a crawl.

So, we need to keep our vehicles "tuned up" and running, just like our metabolism. If we keep our metabolism running, then it will use the stored energy (or fat) more effectively. This continuous use of energy keeps the vehicle that we live in more efficient when it comes to cleaning our systems of excess fat. Then, we don't have to watch every single calorie that we put into our mouths. Because if we enjoy those high-calorie foods now and then, and our body is accustomed to burning fat (or fuel), then we don't have to be obsessed with everything that we eat. And, our bodies stay in shape. We look better, and we feel better.

You can train your body to be an efficient machine by burning off excess fat. It may take a little while to get the engine (or metabolism) revved up, but once you do, it will run more efficiently, and using that stored energy will get easier with time. Keep in mind that it is not necessary to overdo it and work out constantly.

The muscles actually need a break to rebuild and grow stronger. So, even if you start exercising a couple of times per week, it can really help to balance your weight. And, it becomes another effective tool for good health over the course of your life.

Exercising Can Connect Mind and Body

Getting some exercise is not only good for our bodies, it's also good for our minds. The mind-body connection cannot be understated. For example, when a person is depressed, they may not feel like exercising, but if they can just get themselves moving, it can actually help to relieve their depression. Physical activity can change our brain chemistry, which can affect how we think and feel. In a similar way, our thoughts can affect our body's responses. As a result, you can train your body to train your mind, and the other way around.

And, in many ways, getting some exercise feeds our soul. As we get involved in physical activities that we enjoy, it also helps us to re-connect with who we really are. Exercise is also a great way to alleviate stress. If you have difficulty sleeping, it can help you to sleep more deeply so that you can function better physically and mentally.

Remember the fun you had as a child? The focus back then had to do with playing and having a good time. And, of course, that did not involve food, drugs, alcohol, or anything else that could be used in excess. The addictive behaviors that are sometimes used by adults to alleviate stress or certain emotional issues, is detrimental to their health and well-being.

Our busy adult lives can sometimes get the best of us. We become so involved in our day-to-day responsibilities, that we lose that sense of fun that we once had as a child when we ran and played. As a result, our weight may have become out of balance. Our health may be adversely affected, and our stress levels most likely increased. We may not be getting the amount of sleep that we got as a child when we were "worn out" after a busy day of playing.

What can you do now? Start by thinking of something that you enjoyed doing at one time. Some people enjoy going to a gym and/or having a trainer work with them, while other people enjoy other ways to exercise, such as riding a bike, taking a walk in a park, or perhaps getting into a team sport.

Was there a type of sport that you enjoyed when you were younger? If so, is there a way that you can get back into doing that sport with some friends? Are there any groups in your area that get together to enjoy that type of activity? If not, then maybe you can start your own group. Just imagine how helpful that could be not only to yourself, but to many others. (Some women have had success at Curves fitness centers, where they connect with other women by working out in a circle.)

The group setting is a great way to make friends, and to possibly find some support in what you are doing. This support can inspire us to keep going, and not give up on the activity. These groups can provide us with a connection to other people that can be healing in many ways. The end result is stress relief for our minds, physical fitness for our bodies, and emotional healing for our souls.

Whether it is an exercise group, or some physical activity that is done with a group, finding a group of people that are of similar size can create a sense of connection. Chances are you will feel more comfortable with that group, since you will most likely have more in common with them. But if a group is not what you are looking for, there are many activities that can provide both fun and fitness.

Dancing can be allot of fun, and can really get your heart pumping. If you don't have a partner, there are dance groups that get into all types of dancing from Ballroom to Jazz or Tango to Country-Western.

Feeling adventuresome? You can check out the rock-climbing wall, either at your local gym or at places that have just indoor rock climbing. For something less daring, you can find hiking trails online. The trails are often rated for difficulty. And, all you need is a comfortable pair of hiking boots and a small pack for water and snacks.

Along the lines of hiking is a sport called Geocaching (geochacing.com). It's kind of like treasure hunting, only you use a hand-held GPS unit to locate a "cache" that contains various small items such as souvenirs, foreign coins, or anything small (but not edible) that can be put into a weather-proof container.

Often-times these "caches" are placed in a picturesque area, or can lead you to a place that you did not know existed. It can be a good family game that involves some hiking, as the kids learn about geographical coordinates, while they are out in nature. Some of them are "urban caches" that are located in a city park, or somewhere in town.

There are caches all over the world, and information on approximate location and coordinates can be found on the website where you can print the information out and take it with you. (Clues as to where the cache is hidden are also on the website.) So if you are going on vacation, why not go on a little treasure hunt?

There are also "travel bugs," which are small items that can be located in a cache that have a dog tag with a number. The travel bug has its own identification number, and is on a "mission" to go to some specific destination. People can help the travel bug to get to where it is going by taking it and putting it in another cache, so that it will get closer to its final destination. This is just another fun game to play that can help families to get outdoors and get some exercise.

You can learn something new like taking surfing lessons or skiing lessons. Maybe you have always wanted to learn gymnastics, or some other sport. The activity of learning something new can really help us to take our mind off of our problems, plus stimulate our brain cells.

If you find an activity that you really enjoy, you will have a tendency to stick with it longer. And even though it may not be a high fat burning activity, if you have a tendency to do it more often, then it can be very effective for weight management. But if you prefer variety, it is a great idea to "mix it up" by trying different things.

If none of these ideas interest you, then simply taking a walk can help relieve stress, and can also take us away from focusing on food as a stress-reliever. Rather than using comfort food, why not find comfort by walking in nature? Breathing in some fresh air and enjoying the beauty of the outdoors can be very relaxing for our mind, and is healthful for our bodies.

Some people enjoy taking their dogs for a walk, which benefits both them and their pet. There are other people who enjoy seeing wild animals such as bird-watching, or taking a walk around their local zoo. (Many zoos have annual memberships, which can save money for those people who like to visit the zoos often.) And, looking at animals can have a stress relieving affect, because it takes our minds off of our worries and cares.

Other Aspects of Exercise

Let's look at another aspect of exercise. When we think of aerobics, we think of having to do allot of jumping around and sweating. But the word aerobics has to do with providing oxygen to the body. After all, oxygen is needed to help burn excess fat. And, sometimes we forget to take a few deep breaths, which we need to feed our bodies, and to relax our minds.

One possibility is yoga. Yoga involves stretching and breathing for health and well-being. However it is important to start slow, and work your way up to more strenuous levels of yoga. Some people attempt to go beyond their capabilities in the beginning, which can pull a muscle or two. So, it is good to take it slow and enjoy the gradual process. Yoga can help us to connect mind, body and soul, and helps us to realize that we are all connected to one another.

There are even breathing exercises (such as Bodyflex) that can take inches off of peoples bodies. The exercise involves simply stretching and breathing, which can be helpful for those people who are unable to get up and walk around (such as people who are in a wheelchair). So you see, it is possible to burn some excess fat even if you are not able to use your muscles.

If you are able to use your muscles (especially your legs, and particularly the thighs, since that is where the larger muscles are), then you can use those muscles to burn fat. As I said at the beginning of the chapter, muscle is like the engine of the body, and fat is like stored fuel (or energy), it is important to keep that metabolism going by maintaining muscle. After all, a pound of muscle burns approximately 40 calories per day. Which means that five pounds of muscle burns about 200 calories per day, (even when you are not getting exercise). In other words, maintaining muscle can allow you to eat more, and still maintain a body that is physically fit.

This helps to take the focus off of "dieting." Especially since many diets often result in deprivation — and that's no fun. Not to mention that restrictive eating actually slows down the metabolism, where as exercise increases the metabolism.

Here is a technical thought: Regular exercise, especially resistance training, stimulates thyroid hormone secretions and increases tissue sensitivity to the hormone, raising basal metabolism. In other words, when you increase muscle mass your body begins to burn more fat.

Some of the weight loss ads on TV, in magazines or newspapers, often show people with their before and after photos. And although the ad is for a weight loss pill or some type of diet, it is clear in the after picture that the person has developed some muscle, because they look firm and toned. Sometimes the muscle development is very obvious.

You know the saying: "if you don't use it, you'll lose it." It's true with our bodies. As people age, if they do not get some regular exercise, the average person can gain about one and a half pounds of fat each year, while they lose one half pound of muscle each year.

When it comes down to simply getting some exercise, a stationary bike may work for some people, especially if they have a habit of watching certain television shows, or they are really into reading. In other words, if you are going to sit and watch television or read, why not sit on a stationary bicycle? Next thing you know, a half hour will be gone and you just burned some excess fat while building muscle. And once you make it a habit, you will actually miss doing it. (Kind of like brushing your teeth.) Although, keep in mind that it generally takes at least three weeks to create a habit.

The most effective way to build muscle and burn fat is through progressive resistance training. This can be done inexpensively by purchasing a set of elastic bands that provide different levels of weight through resistance. One brand is Bodylastics (bodylastics.com).

Their set of elastic bands comes with an instruction booklet, and can be purchased with a DVD.

It is good to "mix up" the workout for variety. And, it has been shown that doing 15 minutes of endurance training (such as running on a treadmill) and 15 minutes of strength training (which can be with resistance or dumbbells) is more effective than just endurance training alone.

It should also be mentioned that in some ways, less is more. Training too much is actually not as effective as when you give your body a chance to recover in between, because the body has to have a chance to build muscle and repair. Studies have shown that over time, working out two days per week (with a couple of days in between workouts) has the same benefit as working out for three days per week.

You should rest at least three days, and at the most seven days between exercise sessions. And after the first two weeks of "breaking in", never train more than twice weekly. It all goes back to balance and moderation (with both exercise *and* eating).

You can also try to increase your activity whenever or wherever there is an opportunity to do so. If you sit at a desk all day, you can make a point of getting up and walking around every now and then. If there is an area where you can walk near your work, you could spend some time on your lunch hour going for a walk. If there are some stairs and you are able to take a break, you could go for a walk up and back down the stairs. (Especially if you are feeling stressed or you need a break from the boss or co-worker.)

The thigh muscles are some of the largest muscles in the body, which means they burn more calories than most other muscles. One of the simplest ways to exercise is to bend the knees, and do a few squats. You can do that while you brush your teeth, or if you are standing near a counter top, or next to something that you can hold on to while you squat down, and stand up. It's amazing how simple it can be to build some muscle, and tone our bodies.

Free Yourself from the Scale

As people age, they can maintain the same weight, while actually becoming larger. They can find that they do not wear the same size of clothing as they did when they were younger. This is because a pound of muscle takes up about 20 percent less space than a pound of fat. This is one reason why a better way of keeping track of how you are doing is by taking body measurements, rather than using a scale. Also, muscle has a firm shape, supports the body, and helps maintain good posture. On the other hand, fat sags and drags the body downward.

Keep in mind that muscle weighs more than fat. This is another reason why the scale is not an affective measure of fitness. When you begin to build muscle and lose fat, you can actually gain a couple of pounds, while your body measurements decrease. Remember that this is not the time to get discouraged (thinking that you are putting on weight). Gaining muscle is a good thing, because that muscle will continue to burn excess fat, even when you are not getting any exercise.

As hard as it may seem to give up the scale, it can be better for us in the long run, both mentally and physically. Since we are all built differently (with a different muscle mass and bone density), a person may not be able to reach as low a weight as someone else. So by avoiding the scale, we can actually feel better about ourselves, because we are not busy comparing our weight with others. After all, it is possible that we may never weigh what someone in a magazine weighs.

And when you start to look more fit, then you can begin to feel better about yourself. This renewed sense of self can be very motivating. Once you see the results, then it can inspire you to become even more fit. Next thing you know, you have created a good habit. But to really see the results, you can start to measure from the very beginning.

To take body measurements, all you need is a flexible measuring tape (either cloth or plastic) and a piece of paper. Wearing either thin clothes (or no clothes at all), measure yourself in front of a mirror so that you can see if you have the measuring tape in the correct place. Make sure your muscles are relaxed, and pull the tape together (but not too tight, so as not to stretch the tape). On the following page is a diagram of a body and where you can measure to track your changing shape.

There are five places that you can measure: The chest, biceps, waist, hips and thigh. (Remember to measure the same arm or thigh each time.) The *chest* measurement should be around the largest part of the chest. Measure your *bicep* between your elbow and up to the top part of your shoulder. The *waist* is measured in the narrowest part, or about one inch above the navel. The *hips* should be measured with your feet together, and around the largest area. And finally the *thigh* is also measured in the largest part. While you are getting some form of exercise, try measuring yourself once per week, instead of getting on the scale. You may appreciate those results more.

It's good to keep in mind that as we age, it can get harder to take up some type of physical activity. In other words, if someone is doing a physical activity at the age of 80, chances are they have been doing it for a while. That person is more likely able to manage their weight and stay healthier as they age. And, they are actually having fun doing it, because it is probably something that they *enjoy* doing. So why put off a healthy habit? There is no time like the present.

It may help to think about the health benefits of physical activity (besides the fat burning capabilities). Getting some exercise can help lower cholesterol, balance blood sugar (and the way the body handles sugar), it can positively affect brain cells (like when we sleep), and improve the overall metabolism of the body.

More Benefits of Exercise

When people who are physically fit eat sugar, it is sent directly to the muscle instead of being stored as fat. (Because the body of a fit person is used to needing the energy for when they exercise.) When the sugar is sent to the muscle, it is burned more quickly and easily. So being fit can give you some leeway in your ability to eat sugar. After all, who wants to go through life never eating any sugar at all?

The fitness level of the body can also have a positive affect on cholesterol. After cholesterol is eaten, it eventually goes to the liver where it is wrapped in protein. In a fit body, the liver has a tendency to wrap more protein around the cholesterol. The result is HDL (high density lipo-protein) which is better than LDL (low density lipo-protein) because it sinks in the blood.

The effect of physical activity on the brain is that people can go into a deeper level of sleep (such as R.E.M. sleep). The end result is that you can get the same amount of sleep in less time. Also, you will feel more rested, and your overall ability to think clearly and focus will improve. Exercise can also increase endorphins in the brain. These endorphins can help us handle stress, and make us feel better mentally.

Exercising helps to increase the body's metabolic rate (improving metabolism) since muscles need fat for energy. However when it comes to the body's ability to burn fat, the truth is that the body needs some fat, some sugar and some oxygen. They all work together for effective excess fat burning. Once again, balance is the best thing.

Review of Benefits

With your chosen activity (or activities), you can create a sense of well-being. You may form new friendships that can provide support. You may renew some happy memories of the fun you once had when you were younger. Physically, you will enjoy your fit body with its better balance and stamina.

You may notice certain health benefits that can positively affect your heart, cholesterol or blood sugar. You may find that you are sleeping better. Mentally, you will reduce your level of stress, and you may feel more emotionally balanced. Your activity can provide nourishment for your soul, and ultimately a re-connection with who you really are.

7

No Pain, No Gain

History, despite its wrenching pain, cannot be unlived, however, if faced with courage, need not be lived again.

— **Maya Angelou**

The saying "no pain, no gain" is generally used to describe muscle soreness from working out. However, in this case the term refers to emotional healing and its positive effect on weight. The way that a person thinks and feels can have a major impact on their weight.

Unfortunately, negative emotions can cause overeating. Perhaps we are mad at our spouse, so we eat out of anger. Sometimes our internal emotions get the best of us, and we can wind up "stuffing" that emotion with food. Or, we eat when we are alone, to comfort ourselves. Sometimes we feel exhausted from stress or lack of sleep, and we have the desire to eat in order to feel more energetic. If we are not getting enough rest, then we may grab a few sweets for some "quick energy."

It is possible a person's excess weight can be a reflection of the pain that they carry inside. There may be subconscious reasons why a person over-eats, and they probably are not consciously aware of the underlying reason. For example, someone who has been molested may eat to gain weight so they will be less attractive. Whatever the reason, when a person decides to diet they can become more unhappy and frustrated, which causes them to wind up over-eating again and gain even more weight.

Hunger is the body's need for nourishment, controlled by the levels of nutrients in the blood. However, hunger is not the only reason we eat. How much and what we ate at our last meal, our eating schedule, the climate (since heat can make us less hungry and cold can make us more hungry), exercise (which can increase our hunger), our hormone levels, and any illnesses that we may be experiencing can affect what and how we eat. When we want to eat but are not hungry, then we just have an appetite (or craving).

An appetite is our *desire* to eat rather than the *need* to eat. This desire can be caused by either positive or negative emotions, thoughts, memories, sights and smells and types of food (foods high in sugar, fat or salt). Naturally, people have a tendency to look for the maximum amount of energy in the easiest way possible, which is why people are drawn to fast food.

Sometimes we are hungry, but have no appetite (especially when we are ill). Humans were naturally designed to eat the correct amount of food. However, today we don't listen to our bodies. Our appetite controls us instead of us controlling our appetite and we eat without being hungry.

When we are hungry, we should eat only until we are satisfied. Remember, that it takes about 20 minutes for the brain to realize that the stomach is full. It, therefore, is best to eat slowly. However, it is a good idea not to allow ourselves to get *too* hungry, because we will be more likely to over-eat. As I have said before, five small meals each day is often recommended, because it keeps the metabolism going, and you won't become overly hungry. Snacking can be a good thing. Again, it's just about finding balance, and not eating for emotional reasons.

In the case of the occasional treat, such as having a piece of birthday cake or some other situation where we choose to partake in something that we truly enjoy, that's fine. We should enjoy it, without over-indulging to the point of binge-eating. It always goes back to moderation.

Do Emotions Control Your Eating?

If you are not hungry, and you eat anyway, ask yourself why. Most often a person is simply not aware of what is driving them to overeat. Usually the person who is eating for emotional reasons, will eat as soon as they get home from work, and whenever they are bored. The person will suddenly feel hungry, as if they are instantly starving, and have to eat right now. But it is important to remember that real hunger is gradual. Hunger manifests through a growling stomach that may come and go over a couple of hours. You may feel that you need to eat soon, but there is a sense of patience. Hunger is not a craving for a specific food, as is the case with an emotional appetite, where a person feels they've got to have potato chips, or chocolate, etc.

Is the desire to eat coming from your taste desire rather than your stomach? If so, it may be emotional rather than physical hunger. The emotional eater can feel uncomfortable talking about their feelings, and food is used to calm those feelings instead of expressing them. As a result, they may feel hungry almost all of the time, because the emotions are still there, since they are not being expressed.

Eating emotionally often occurs after something upsetting has happened, rather than when a person feels a physical need to eat. Not paying attention to what you are eating is another sign of emotional eating. When you eat large amounts of food without realizing it, it is an indication that you are eating for emotional reasons.

If you are eating to make yourself feel better, but become angry with yourself or feel guilty about eating, you are eating out of emotion. You then create even more negative emotions, and the vicious cycle of over-eating continues.

Becoming Aware

In the case of emotional eating, it is important to think about when it all began. Was there a divorce or the loss of a loved one? Or perhaps some other situation occurred to begin to try to fill the emptiness with food. Unfortunately, food will never completely satisfy the emptiness that a person may be feeling. Using food for comfort can backfire and actually be the cause behind obesity.

The over-eating of certain foods can indicate what is going on in a person's life. Studies have shown that when a person is stressed, the brain hormones may cause the person to crave salty pretzels. Loneliness can lead to wanting crackers and pasta. Anxiety can make a person crave soft sweet foods like ice cream. Depression can create a desire to eat sweets. If a person is angry, they may feel the need to eat meat or crunchy foods. Jealousy can cause someone to want to eat large quantities of just about anything.

A slight change in the brain hormones can cause someone to be highly emotional, and lead them to over-eat. Too much or too little of a brain hormone can cause serious health problems.

Sit down and think about when you were a child. We may have developed a habit of comforting ourselves that began when we were children. Maybe our mother gave us a treat when we "skinned our knee," or just felt unhappy. This can trigger our subconscious mind to treat ourselves to feel better. When this begins early in life, it can seem a difficult habit to resolve, but it can be done.

Look Inside Yourself

Rather than worrying about what you are eating, pay attention to the emotions and what is going on — on the inside. When you become aware that you need to comfort yourself with food, try to use a journal to write down your thoughts and emotions. Are you depressed, frustrated, angry or lonely? Is there some other reason that you have a craving? Express your feelings in your journal, rather than expressing them by eating. If there is a "hole" that needs to be filled, find out what that "hole" is.

Becoming aware of why we are eating, and the emotions behind it, can help us to connect with ourselves. When we feel disconnected with our true self, it becomes difficult to identify our emotions. As a result, depression can set in, along with a feeling of hopelessness. Then we become disconnected from our mind and are not aware of what is really going on inside. We are not "conscious" of how our emotions are affecting our body.

It is best to slow down, and quietly look inward. See where any negative emotions may be coming from. Sometimes we eat a particular food because it brings back a memory of our childhood. For example, our parents or grandparents cheered us up with a cookie when we were feeling sad. Understanding this, we can learn to let go of negative thoughts and emotions with something other than food.

Again, use your journal to write down how you feel before, during, and after you have finished eating. By doing this, you can become more conscious of what is going on inside, and not just what is happening on the outside. If you feel a craving, take a deep breath, and take a moment to pay attention to your feelings. Close your eyes, and feel where the craving is coming from.

Spend at least a week writing down your feelings, especially when you are having cravings. You will, then, be able to see the source of the negative emotions. When this happens, allow yourself to experience the emotion, rather than trying to comfort the emotion with food. You can continue to write about it, or express your feelings to someone in order to let the emotions out. When you understand what is causing the emotions that are leading to the emotional eating, you can find other ways to deal with the emotion without using food.

You can also write down anyone or anything that has ever been irritating to you, or has simply made you angry. If you cannot remember their name, then just describe who they were to you. You can then say to everyone on the list that you forgive them. If you feel that you cannot forgive them, then at least let go of the connection to them, and release them to the universe, as you take in a deep breath and imagine yourself letting go, and sending them away from you.

By letting negative thoughts go, you take responsibility for yourself, and release any resentment that you may have toward yourself and others. As a result, you will feel better about yourself, which improves your self-esteem, something that is vital in balancing your weight.

Becoming Mindful

As stated previously, we do not want to completely deprive ourselves of the foods we enjoy. But we need to be mindful, and slow down our eating and enjoy it without eating emotionally.

When you are eating, connect what is going on inside with the external environment, and be aware mentally and physically. Being mindful is not being judgmental, but just paying attention. It can free us from habits, and reactive behavior due to emotions. It helps us to feel balanced, and promotes choice. It allows us to become more positive, and to respect our own inner wisdom.

By eating mindfully, we learn to enjoy our food using all of our senses. We can understand our likes and dislikes more by being more aware of our food. It helps us to understand our physical hunger, so that we can notice when we should stop eating.

Each of us is unique. We need to understand our individual needs on a moment-to-moment basis. The focus is on the immediate choices that are made regarding our eating, rather than the distant health outcome from our choices. Being mindful gives us insight into how we can act to achieve our health goals, allowing us to become more empowered with our eating.

Mindful eating has to do with choosing food that involves all of your senses. We should choose food that is nourishing and pleasing. The first steps that we can take toward mindful eating include the following suggestions from The Center for Mindful Eating (TCME):

1. Become *aware* of what is going on *while* you are eating. By using all of your senses, you can enjoy the sights, smells, sounds and textures of your food. You can learn to enjoy each bite more when you really pay attention as you chew your food slowly, and enjoy the flavors and textures.

2. Start to *think* about why you are eating a certain food. Understanding why you chose that food can help you to understand the emotional aspect of eating.

3. Focus on the reason for the *choice*. Why did you choose to eat the foods that you are eating at this time and place? If it is an unhealthy food choice, what drove you to choose that? What

was going on physically, mentally and emotionally? (Remember to exercise self-respect and understanding.)

4. How do those choices about foods *help* or *harm* you. Do your choices affect others such as your spouse and/or children?

You don't need to worry about conquering all of the steps at once. You can start with one meal, or one day to practice just one step. If you begin with the first step, you can use it until you feel comfortable with it, and then you can try the second step.

You can also learn to be "in the moment" or fully present when you eat, rather than being focused on the emotions and binging out of the need for comfort. You can practice with a "mindful meditation," which can allow you to feel more content and centered within yourself.

You can start by putting less food on your plate, knowing that you can take more if you continue to feel hungry after you have finished eating that amount. Sometimes our eyes are "bigger than our stomach," and we end up piling on more than we can comfortably eat. Then we may feel compelled to finish all of the food that we took. Remember it is alright not to eat everything that is on our plate, so don't feel guilty about not finishing all of it.

Chinese monks and nuns use something called an "alms bowl," which is a bowl that is "the instrument for appropriate measure." If the food fills the bowl, then it is considered to be sufficient. Some people eat off of a nine-inch or smaller plate, to try and keep their portions down. However, this is not about starvation or deprivation, but about experiencing joy, satisfaction and contentment with the food that we eat. In doing so, we can avoid the feeling of guilt from overeating or being physically bloated and "overstuffed" when we eat too much food too quickly.

How to Eat Mindfully

When you begin to eat, simply take a small, bite-sized piece of food and put it in your mouth. Now pay attention to that piece of food, and notice how it feels in your mouth. You can feel it on your tongue, and touching the roof of your mouth. As you slowly chew your bite of food, notice the texture of it. Is it soft or crunchy? Is it warm, cold or room temperature? What is the flavor like: Is it sweet, salty, sour or spicy?

Keep chewing the food for at least 30 chews, and notice whether the flavor changes. Does the food liquefy, or does it maintain a shape as you chew it? Does eating this food bring back a pleasant memory? Even though you may be eating something simple like oatmeal, if you are fully in the moment, you can enjoy the tastes and texture of it. When we thoroughly chew our food, it becomes half digested. Then when the food gets to our stomach, it becomes easier to digest, and more nutrients can be absorbed into the body.

While eating mindfully, the chewing of food is for enjoying and appreciating that which was lovingly prepared. Swallow the food, feeling it going down your throat to your stomach, where your hunger gradually becomes satisfied as you slowly continue to eat.

You can practice this mindful meditation as you eat a small meal. By doing so, it can help you to fully appreciate your food, and slow down your eating. Any memories that you may have can allow you to connect with yourself, and you can feel more satisfied.

The same technique for mindful eating can be used for mindful drinking, including when a person consumes alcohol. The drink can be enjoyed slowly, by noticing the smell, taste, and even the color of the beverage. This mindful drinking can help to avoid over-doing it in the case of alcohol consumption.

Changing our Attitude

At times of loneliness, anger, grief, or any other emotion that may cause us to over-indulge, we can begin to change that feeling by using an effective tool known as appreciation. It's surprising how easily we can shift how we feel, from a negative emotion to a positive emotion, by simply changing our perspective. It can happen almost instantly. This attitude of appreciation can be felt while we are slowly chewing and enjoying our food. Feeling appreciative can help us to savor and enjoy the wonderful food that we have.

No matter what happens, there is always hope, and it is always possible to find something to feel good about. If thinking appreciative thoughts work, then do that. But writing it down can work even better. So keep a journal by the bed, or keep it with you during the day and write something positive down. Appreciation is one of the biggest keys to mind-body wellness. By changing your attitude with appreciation, you can reduce the desire for emotional eating.

Use the power of positive thinking. When it comes to eating, if you are trying to not eat something, think about what you are gaining instead of what you are giving up. Instead of saying "I really miss eating a cheeseburger with French fries for lunch," say to yourself "I really enjoyed the healthier sandwich with fruit that I ate for lunch."

We can stay more positive if we pay attention to what is happening around us. Sometimes it is best to avoid negative people. But if that is not possible, then try to change the subject to one that is more positive. Hopefully it will not only make you feel better, but you may be helping the other person feel better as well.

If the television is on and the news or program is depressing, then change it to something that is uplifting and makes you feel good. Watching a comedy can change our mood quickly. Or simply do whatever it is to make yourself feel good inside. By doing so, you can feed your soul, and feel satisfied from the inside out.

Overview

The following is a list of suggestions to help curb emotional eating:

1. *Are you really hungry?* Pay attention to how you feel physically. Is it really hunger, or just a craving?

2. *Know your triggers.* For a few days, write down what you eat, how much, when, how you are feeling when you are eating and how hungry

you are. Also look for patterns. Does the same feeling occur when you over-indulge?

3. *Look elsewhere for comfort.* Find something else to do, such as writing in a journal or going for a walk. Do something you enjoy. Call your "buddy" (someone that is supporting you in your weight management). Write how you feel in your journal. Keep an appreciation log. (Write down things that you are appreciative of — particularly at night before bed, to focus on the positive. This can help to turn your emotions around.)

4. *Don't keep unhealthy foods around.* If the "comfort" foods are not in the house, then it will make it easier to not reach for them in times of stress (or distress). Try not to shop when you are having cravings that are related to emotional eating or fatigue.

5. *Have healthy snacks.* Snack on whole foods. (Foods that are natural, such as fruit, or a few almonds.) As mentioned elsewhere in this book, keep in mind that it takes 60 to 90 days before you may enjoy the taste of natural foods, after snacking on processed, high sugar or high fat foods. But once you become re-sensitized to it, then it will become just as

enjoyable, or perhaps even more enjoyable than those other foods.

6. *Eat in moderation.* As also mentioned previously, it is not necessary to deprive yourself of entire food groups. It's OK to eat some carbs, without going overboard. If you are not getting all of the calories that you need, you can have a tendency to eat more for emotional reasons. So eat regularly, and preferably five smaller meals to keep the metabolism going. You should never feel like you are "starving." It can also help to eat more fiber, like choosing whole grains such as brown rice instead of white rice, and whole grain or sourdough bread instead of white bread.

7. *Eat some breakfast.* There is a reason why it is called: Break-fast. Although the metabolism slows down when we sleep, we need to help get it going after we wake up in the morning. It is a good idea to eat within one hour after waking. Try some oatmeal (preferably low or no sugar). Instead, try adding fruit. Eggs are actually a good way to start the day, and are considered to be relatively lean.

8. *Exercise regularly.* (See the chapter on Fitness for Mind, Body and Soul.)

9. *Get enough sleep.* You will have a tendency to eat healthier if you are getting enough rest. Your metabolism can slow down if you are tired.

There are certain foods that naturally contain ingredients that make us feel better emotionally. Some of those foods are: Chicken, turkey, red meat, dairy products, nuts, seeds, bananas, halibut, shrimp, salmon, snapper, tuna and shellfish. These foods contain tryptophan, which increases the levels of the feel-good hormone serotonin.

Omega-3 fatty acids can boost brain power to help relieve depression. (Studies have also shown that it can also help prevent Alzheimer's disease.) It is contained in the following foods: Albacore tuna, salmon, trout, mackerel, herring and sardines.

Slowing down and becoming aware of our eating, and using techniques (such as journaling and appreciation), in addition to adding wholesome foods throughout the day, can help ease our emotional pain, and avoid the negative affects that emotional eating has on our bodies. These tools can give us the additional support that can help us to find balance in our lives, and re-connect with ourselves.

8

Imagine

Imagination is the beginning of creation. You imagine what you desire, you will what you imagine and at last you create what you will.
— **George Bernard Shaw (1856-1950)**

*M*indfulness eating and other tools for weight management are certainly helpful. They can help us to pay closer attention to what we are doing, so that we can learn to slow down and enjoy. That is what works at the conscious level of the mind. But the subconscious is really the majority (about 88 percent) of our mind, and that is where our habits and emotions are. And quite often, it is those habits and emotions that overpower our desire to control or change our actions. People may say that you are what you eat. However, you really are what you *think*, and more importantly, how you *feel*. Therefore, true change can occur by unlocking the power of the subconscious mind.

The subconscious mind is on the same level as the soul, which is why it remembers everything. In other words, everything that we have ever experienced in our lives is stored there. This is why we may react to things in a certain way, and do not consciously know why we felt the way we did. Something might happen to us that triggers a memory, and we may react emotionally without having a clue as to why we are feeling a certain way.

It is that sense of feeling disconnected from ourselves, or our soul, that can result in the inability to resolve an issue. That issue may include gaining an unhealthy amount of weight, or it may be the inability to let go of the weight that we are "holding on" to. But when there is connection, there is understanding. And when we understand the situation, we can resolve the problem.

To better understand what is going on at the subconscious level, we need to understand how the mind works. We may not realize it, but it is the subconscious mind that programs us, because we react to things based on our past experience. We develop habits that seem to control us because we have been programmed to react a certain way. For example, we may have developed a habit to eat a certain food at a certain time of day. It is a habit that can be difficult to overcome.

We get our sense of intuition and inspiration from the subconscious mind, which is believed by some people to come from a spiritual level. It is believed that when we are in an altered state of consciousness, we can actually gain insight from other "dimensions." Being in an altered state of consciousness is something we do naturally and regularly. For instance when we sleep, day-dream or go through biochemical changes in our body (such as fevers, or perhaps drugs) we enter into altered states of consciousness.

Actually, we are continually shifting in an out of this altered state throughout the day. For example, have you ever driven home from work, and after arriving home you barely remember driving? You may think to yourself, "I don't really remember the trip home," but you were still able to function even though your mind was drifting in and out of a daydream.

Also, when we watch television, we enter into an altered state of consciousness, becoming lost in the sights and sounds of the story that we are watching. During the day, we can actually use "day dreaming" to help us to reach a goal.

People may refer to it as Visualization, Guided Imagery or Guided Meditation.

The subconscious uses stories or imagery to identify an experience, and we can actually create positive change in our lives by giving our mind a story that it can relate to. We can do this with the use of guided imagery (or guided meditation), which is using our imagination in order to accomplish a particular goal, or to release unresolved issues that may be buried at the subconscious level of the mind.

It was Albert Einstein who said: "Imagination is more important than knowledge." It is our imagination that gives us ideas and inspiration. When we sleep we are at the subconscious level of the mind, and our dreams are part of our imagination. Dreams are a metaphor, or a story, that are symbolic of something else. We can achieve our goals — or dreams by creating a metaphor that relates to the goal we want to reach.

For example, if your goal is to reach your ideal weight, you might close your eyes and imagine seeing yourself in the mirror at your ideal weight. You can then imagine that you are stepping into the mirror and merging with that image. Finally, imagine stepping out of that mirror as you remain at that ideal weight, feeling healthy and confident.

In 1937, Napoleon Hill published a book titled *Think and Grow Rich*. The book was the result of 20 years of research and interviewing successful men including Henry Ford, Andrew Carnegie, Charles Schwab, Theodore Roosevelt, John D. Rockefeller and Thomas Edison. Included in the book is a chapter on the power of the subconscious mind as it relates to reaching a goal. Mr. Hill stated that "there is plenty of evidence to support the belief that the subconscious mind is the connecting link between the finite mind of man and Infinite Intelligence." He also said that the subconscious mind is the tool that is used to pray through, reaching the source that is able to answer the prayer.

Even at that time, Mr. Hill recognized that the subconscious mind is always working, and to reach a goal we need to give it a thought to focus on. And it is not just about thoughts, but also emotions, because our emotions are at the subconscious level. So it is important to create positive thoughts with positive emotions, to feed our subconscious mind (and our soul) so that we really can achieve our goals.

Mr. Hill discussed the power of Auto-Suggestion, which is like an affirmation (see the chapter on Re-Connecting with Yourself for information on affirmations). He also discussed the power of the imagination, and that it was the "fifth step to riches" and "the workshop of the mind." He said that man's only limitation is the lack of the use of his (or her) imagination.

Early on, some of the information was not published in the book because it was perceived to be too controversial. However, more recently the information has been included in unabridged additions of the book, and once again the power of human imagination has come to the surface as a viable tool for success.

When it comes to weight, people should begin to understand the imbalance from the conscious level of the mind. They could ask themselves if they are hungry. In the case of over-eating, the answer would probably be "no." But the real question becomes: Why am I craving? What is going on at the subconscious level of the mind that is creating an empty hole that is not being filled? Discover the answer to that, and a positive change can take place. There are various techniques that can help us create success through the most power tool: Our imagination

First of all, whatever we focus on in the mind, is generally what the body will do. This is why athletes use visualization to imagine playing their sport successfully, and that can ultimately improve their performance. For example, they may imagine successfully shooting basketballs through a hoop. And amazingly, it can actually help their goal-scoring ability.

At the same time, it is important to not have too many goals, but rather to be focused in one area at a time. And, using visualization should be fun and enjoyable. If it feels like a chore, then it may not work for us. So it is important to relax and enjoy the process.

A suggestion is to simply take a few minutes to relax and get in touch with your inner self. You might imagine being in a peaceful place that allows you to feel content and connected to the earth. Imagine that a white light surrounds you and protects you each day, helping you to feel safe and secure within yourself. This sense of security can also help you to feel balanced, without the need to fill an emptiness with excess food.

Feel relaxed with your eyes closed, allow yourself to feel safe and protected. Imagine that you feel nurtured, choosing to take care of yourself. Realize that you are special in every way, as you continue to feel relaxed and peaceful. While you feel surrounded by the soothing white light, you become more empowered to take control of your life, understanding how important it is to love yourself. This type of meditation can be practiced any time. Just take a moment to become more aware of the connection between the body, mind and soul.

Through the ages, the power of the mind, particularly at the subconscious level has been recognized as a force for positive change, and hypnotherapy has become a tool for positive transformation. With hypnotherapy, the gap between body, mind and soul are bridged. The techniques that are used in hypnotherapy can aid in physical, emotional and spiritual healing.

A hypnotherapist can work with you to effectively facilitate the changes that will help you to achieve and maintain a healthy weight. A hypnotherapist is someone who can help us to relax and reach an altered state of consciousness — or the subconscious mind. This helps us to make the changes that we need to make more quickly than we could do on our own. The hypnotherapist can personalize your sessions, and provide tools that will help you to reach your goal.

The hypnotherapist actually facilitates the process. In other words, all hypnosis is self-hypnosis, as there is no "telling" someone what to do, but assisting them in creating the results that they desire to achieve. (The person is not being controlled or "forced" into an altered state of consciousness.)

The word "hypnos" is the Greek word for sleep, as we can access the subconscious mind while in a relaxed state. In Greek Mythology, *Hypnos* is the god of sleep. From the days of the ancient Greek sleep temples, to the more current era of the Law of Attraction and books about the power of intention, people have continued to recognize the vast power of the imagination.

We can use our imagination to release negative emotions that may be causing emotional eating. Sometimes we want to hold on to things, especially when we have lost someone close to us. This need to "hold on" can result in our need to hold on to weight. Letting go is an emotional relief, and at the same time, we can begin to release that excess weight that we have been holding on to.

When using your imagination, it is important to remember that the mind does not process negatives. It's kind of like the mind of a child. You see, a child does not develop a conscious

mind until about the age of seven. In other
words, they are living at the level of the
subconscious mind. Perhaps this is also why
children have such an active imagination. So if
you say to a child "don't run in the house," they
will do it anyway because they have imagined
doing it, and did not imagine *not* doing it.

Remember to use positive words, such as in
the case of creating a statement that is a goal for
yourself. You can say the statement to yourself,
or post it where you will see it. Again, when it
comes to the subconscious mind, positive
suggestions in the present tense are what works.
Stating that you are "free" of the excess weight is
an example of a positive statement.

Today it is understood that the law of
attraction brings to light the mind can affect our
entire life. The concept is that we attract what
occurs in our life through our thoughts and
emotions. It is the universe that is reacting to our
thoughts, rather than our thoughts being the
result of what is occurring around us.

So it is important to keep in mind that once
again, we can empower ourselves to make the
changes that we need to make. We are not
simply the victims of what happens to us. Once
we recognize that and begin to think and feel

more positive, while focusing on the results instead of what we don't want, then we can transform and re-connect with who we truly are.

We can apply this concept to weight management. We can imagine ourselves slimming down to our ideal weight (or in the case of being too thin, we can imagine being at a healthier weight). And we can not only imagine it, but also feel the positive emotions of what it would be like to already be there. For example, you can imagine seeing yourself in the mirror at a healthy weight, feeling relaxed and confident. Or if you like being at the beach, you can imagine seeing your reflection in the water.

Then you can imagine yourself going into the mirror (or that reflection in the water), becoming that image, and noticing how comfortable you feel. When you step out of that imaginary mirror (or water), you remain as that image you saw. You can repeat this visualization to help you become what you imagine yourself to be. There are many other visualization techniques out there that can help you to reach your goal of a healthy weight. These techniques can be learned in group sessions or workshops, guided meditation CDs or from working one-on-one with a hypnotherapist.

Some people have a learning style that is very visual. In that case, or for that matter for anyone, a vision board can be a great tool. What is it that you need and desire? Whatever that picture may be for you, you can draw it or find and cut a picture out of a magazine. You can also use positive words on your vision board. If you are not sure what you want, then think about how you feel. It's like the saying "go with your gut" (which is once again your subconscious). If it feels good to you, then it is probably the way you should go.

When you have your pictures and/or words, you can put them on a cork bulletin board, in a frame, or wherever you will more often see them. The pictures and words can be changed every now and then to reflect your needs and desires. You can get creative and make a collage of pictures. Simply use a glue stick, and put the pictures on some colored paper. You can also create a vision board on your computer. A website that can help you to create a vision board is: www.visionboardsite.com.

Whether you are a visual person or not, you can get a little creative with your vision board. Then when you look at it, you can not only *see* but *feel* the positive emotions of already having accomplished your goal.

It is also important to believe in yourself, and to know that you are worthy of whatever that desire is that you want. If you can allow yourself to imagine and believe, you will be surprised at what manifests.

Tools for Using Your Imagination

Recline into a comfortable position and with relaxing music in the background. Allow yourself to go into a daydream state to help you visualize or imagine. Another tool that is used to relax is taking in some deep breaths and progressively relaxing every part of your body from your head to your toes. You can also allow yourself to ignore any sounds that are going on around you, as you relax into your own comfortable world.

Imagine yourself the way you would like to be. Keep in mind that you should think of yourself as already reaching your goal. If you imagine that it will happen at some point in the future, then the change may not take place. It must be in the present tense. It's like the old saying "tomorrow never comes."

This relaxed daydreaming state can be done for a few minutes each day, in order to help to inspire the subconscious mind. The result is the ability to re-program our mind so that we can release old habits, and allow ourselves to make the changes that we need to make. It can help us to get "un-stuck" from the rut that we may find ourselves in, and that includes our old unhealthy eating patterns.

Some people listen to guided meditations, which can have soothing music, and/or nature sounds along with someone with a relaxing voice that guides them through some creative imagery. The meditations with guided imagery can be for various goals such as weight, smoking, career success, or whatever the person's goal may be. Guided meditation that gives self-esteem a positive boost is most important, because low self-esteem can often be at the core of why we are not achieving the results that we want in our life.

As you use your imagination to reach your goal, it is important to avoid any negative self-talk. This may seem difficult at first if you are used to thinking and feeling that way, but looking at life from a more positive perspective can be a catalyst for true change. Seeing the cup as half full rather than half empty is not only a better way to create inspiration in your life, but it also makes life more pleasant and enjoyable. After all, life is a journey, so it is important to enjoy. Life is simply a continual accomplishment, as we take things one step at a time.

Sometimes it helps to listen to inspirational CDs in your car, then you can listen to an author or speaker on a specific topic that you are interested in. That speaker may be talking about improving self-esteem, or inspiring you to reach a goal, for example. After all, if you can listen to music and DJs talking in your daily commute, why not listen to something inspirational? It can help to take your mind off of the stressful drive. And listening during your commute can allow you to fit it into your busy schedule. Also, if you have a long-distance road trip, listening to inspirational CDs can make the trip even more worthwhile.

When it comes to re-connecting, If you have lost someone that you wish to re-connect with, then you can imagine yourself reuniting with them and telling them all of the things that you need to say but did not get a chance to say before they were gone. By re-connecting and resolving what is really bothering us underneath, we can heal the inside of ourselves. The result is that the outside can fall into place naturally.

The chapter "Connecting with Others" mentions a breast cancer study by David Spiegel of Stanford University School of Medicine in which a support group met on a weekly basis for supportive-expressive group therapy. Along with the support of the group, the patients used self-hypnosis techniques. At the end of the year, those patients in the treatment group that used self-hypnosis stated that they experienced half the pain of the patients that were in the control group that did not use the self-hypnosis. This is further evidence that using our imagination can have a positive affect on our bodies.

Below is a self-hypnosis guide that can be used for reaching a healthy weight, easing pain, improving sports performance, or to achieve results in other areas of your life.

Self Hypnosis Guide

Set aside 20 minutes per day and find a quiet, comfortable place where you will be undisturbed. It is best to do this at a time when you are alert. Begin by selecting a positive affirmation, such as one of the following:

- ❀ I am calm, relaxed and peaceful.
- ❀ I am happy, healthy, and at my ideal weight.
- ❀ I feel great and look great.

Close your eyes and take several deep breaths, imagining that all of the tension is draining out of your body. Then choose a visualization, such as one of the following, or a visualization you prefer:

❀ Imagine a sunset; see all the beautiful colors. Watch as the sun sinks below the horizon and the evening stars begin to come out.

❀ Imagine that you are relaxing on the beach, feeling the warm soft sand underneath you as you listen to the waves and smell the fresh sea air.

❀ Imagine that you are relaxing in a beautiful garden or meadow, and the temperature is perfect as you enjoy the sights, smells, sounds and sensations there.

Very slowly, relax each area at a time as you move up through your body. Become aware of your feet, and relax that area. Then bring your awareness up through your ankles, knees, thighs, hips, stomach, chest, shoulders, neck and up into your head behind your eyes, and then to a point above the top of your head. Use this progressive relaxation until you are completely relaxed.

Count yourself down, relaxing even more with each number: Five Four Three Two One, and say to yourself: "I am now in a state of deep relaxation." Whether you are or not, it does not matter as you first begin to do these exercises.

What does matter is that you become comfortable with the process.

Tell yourself how long you are going to be "in" hypnosis (fifteen minutes, twenty minutes, etc.) This teaches you to set your "inner" clock.

Thank yourself for the progress you are making. Think of several examples of good in your life. Be appreciative of what you have. See and feel yourself letting go of "stuff" that no longer serves you by imagining standing under a waterfall or perhaps in the rain, and letting all the negativity, such as negative emotions, being washed way. When you do, tell yourself that each time you are in the shower, any negative things you are holding onto will be washed away.

Repeat your positive affirmation in all three persons:

- ❀ I am calm, relaxed and peaceful.
- ❀ You are calm relaxed and peaceful.
- ❀ (<u>Your Name</u>) is calm, relaxed and peaceful.

Repeat this at least three times. More is better, but less is better than not at all. Tell yourself what a great job you are doing. You <u>are</u> doing a great job. It takes courage to want to change yourself.

When you are in this relaxed state, imagine yourself the way you want to be; feeling confident and looking healthy, and being able to do all of the things you want to do. You can see and *feel* that you are enjoying life, while you are living your affirmation.

After you have spent some time in your relaxed "daydream" state say, "Now I am going to count from one to five. When I open my eyes, I will feel alert and refreshed." Count yourself up: One... Two Three Four Five. If you do this before sleep, you can suggest that on five you will move into a normal and natural sleep, until it is time for you to wake. (You will be setting your mental alarm clock!)

In the book *Quantum Healing* — *exploring the frontiers of mind/body medicine*, Dr. Deepak Chopra states that "memory is more important and more primary than matter," and that "healing is the restoration of memory; the memory of who we really are." He further states that in the case of obesity, "it is distorted memories that recreate the fatty cells." So that even when old cells are replaced with new cells, the fatty cells will continue to be created if we do not improve our mind/body connection.

When it comes to hypnotherapy, regression techniques can allow a person to go back to the past in their mind, in order to help them resolve past hurts that may be causing their weight to be out of balance through emotional eating. These memories could be from a person's childhood, or at some other point in their life. They may not be consciously aware that the memory is "hidden" at the subconscious level, and therefore remains unresolved. When the person imagines going back to the past, it allows them to understand and resolve the experience. By doing so, they can find closure with the past experience so that they can let go of the need to soothe their unresolved emotions with food.

Some people may experience a memory that they believe to be part of a past life. Whether we believe this or not, the experience can still result in healing from an emotional issue. Even if the situation that the person "remembers" is merely a metaphor that was created by the mind while in a dream-like state, does it really matter? In other words, if the thoughts, feelings or images that a person perceives helps them to find "the answer" to their problem and allows them to heal from it, then it can still be a helpful tool to assist them to feel connected — mind, body and soul.

The term "whatever works" comes to mind in the case of using the mind and our imagination to achieve healthy results for our bodies. Whether it is using a vision board, guided imagery or guided meditation, regression techniques or whatever works, people can use their imagination to improve their life. Our imagination can help us to find the answer within ourselves, so that we can once again find balance, and transform our lives for the better.

9

Release

Courage is the power to let go of the familiar.
— **Raymond Lindquist**

The answer to weight management is not in a pill. The answer is not contained in some frozen low calorie meal. It is not in some special weight plan sponsored by a movie or television star. The answer is inside you. You hold the key.

Take a look at what is going on inside of yourself and you can find the "answer." Then, a domino affect occurs, and everything begins to fall into place (including your weight). There are various ways you can release and resolve whatever is going on inside yourself that could be affecting your weight.

Part of releasing/letting go involves people taking responsibility for themselves. When someone blames others for their problems, they

147

become disempowered. They are unable to make changes in their life because they believe that someone else has power over them. But when people change their focus from and blame on someone else, and instead focus on themselves, they are enabled with the power to take control of their lives and make some positive changes.

Barbara Walters, when interviewing Oprah Winfrey, asked: "what's the reason you put yourself on the line week after week, year after year, on the cutting edge of human emotion?" Oprah answered: "Teaching people to take responsibility. I believe the secret to life is to take responsibility. Once people grasp that, I believe everything in their life changes. Once people understand it and live it, they are at cause for their life rather than living in effect and reaction."

It is important to ask yourself:

- ☐ How you *feel* when you have the need to eat, even though you are not hungry.
- ☐ What happened in the past that triggered the eating?
- ☐ Is it at a certain time of day, and if so, why?
- ☐ Is it when you are alone?
- ☐ Is there an unresolved emotion that is being bottled up inside?

Releasing and letting go of whatever is being held inside of us, can allow us to let go of the weight and eat more normally.

Through journaling, you may have discovered what triggers you to over-eat. When you know what causes you to eat (such as stress or for emotional reasons) you can use your imagination to let go of the cause of the eating. Or, even if you have not been able to determine the exact cause at a conscious level, you can imagine that you are letting go of whatever may be bothering you at the subconscious level of your mind. In other words, it may be a feeling that you are holding on to, or you might not even be aware of anything at all, since it could be "buried."

You can practice releasing the emotions by closing your eyes and imagining that you are holding a group of balloons of various colors. Each balloon holds a negative emotion such as fear, anger, guilt or sadness. As you release each balloon, imagine that you are letting go of that negative emotion. When you release the underlying cause of the eating, then a transformation can take place.

By bringing the memory that is contained in our bodies at the subconscious level to the conscious level of the mind, we can better understand why we are behaving the way that we do (including our eating habits). By releasing the issues from the past, we can heal the present, and create health benefits for ourselves in the future.

Another way to release any negative emotions that you have been holding on to is simply write a letter to someone (even yourself). By writing your thoughts and emotions down and expressing how you feel, you can let go of negative feelings that you may have been holding on to. You can then dispose of the letter in whatever way helps you to let go of the memories, so that you can move on and feel a sense of acceptance. Resolving those past experiences frees us from "stuffing our feelings."

There are other tools to consider in the case of emotions and weight management. One of the emotions that people try to "stuff" with food is anger. (The emotion of anger is common in the case of eating disorders.) Instead of stuffing the anger with food, why not channel the anger into doing exercise? Take up kickboxing, or any form of exercise in which you can let go of your anger. Sometimes just going for a walk (or run if you are able to) can help you to let go of what is bothering you. After awhile, you may hardly remember what it was that you were upset about. In doing so, you will avoid the added calories while you burn a few calories. In the end, you will feel better; mentally, physically and emotionally.

Crying is Good

Remember that it is OK to express your emotions. The act of crying can help us to get in touch with our feelings, and crying can actually be good for us. It has been proven that emotionally induced tears help to relieve stress by helping us to release potentially harmful chemicals from our body. (These tears have a higher protein content than tears that occur due to eye irritation.)

All animals that live on earth (as opposed to water) produce tears, which lubricates their eyes. But it is only humans that have the ability to cry, and this crying allows people to deal with emotional problems. Scientists have discovered that after crying, people feel better, both physically and psychologically. Without crying, they can actually feel *worse*.

Evidence shows that people feel better after crying, because their body has released toxic substances through their tears. In fact, the type of tears that are produced from watching a sad movie are chemically different from the tears that are produced from slicing an onion. (The tears produced from watching sad movies contain much more toxic biological byproducts.) It was discovered that the crying process removes toxic substances from the body that can build up during times of stress.

Tears from crying contain the following ingredients:

1. Manganese: A mineral which affects mood, and is 30 times higher in concentration in a person's tears than it is in their bloodstream.

2. The protein albumin.

3. Leucine-enkephalin: An endorphin that helps control pain.

4. Poloactin: A hormone that regulates milk production in mammals.

5. Adrenocorticotrophic hormone (ACTH): A chemical compound that is an indicator of stress.

Suppressing tears can increase stress levels, which can contribute to stress-related diseases such as high blood pressure, peptic ulcers and heart problems. Since men in our society are discouraged from crying, they can actually be more vulnerable to stress-related diseases. (Perhaps that is one reason why women generally live longer than men.) There are some people who suffer from an inherited disease called familial dysautonomia, which means that they are physically unable to cry. They also have a very low ability to deal with various stressful situations in their life.

One report suggests that people with stress-related illnesses cry less than people who are healthier. A study was done with 100 men and women with stress-related disorders. 50 had ulcers, and 50 had colitis. They were compared with 50 healthy people who were the same age and had similar life circumstances. The people who had the stress-related disorders believed that crying was a sign of weakness or a loss of control. Those people who were ill were less likely to cry in various situations.

Crying not only allows us to get in touch with our emotions, it also helps us to connect with others. Crying actually helps us to communicate. When you cry, it shows that you are sincere about a certain issue. It fosters a sense of community and concern for other people. Tears can cause those around us to be sympathetic, and crying helps us to bond with others.

Emotional Freedom Technique (EFT)

In the case of emotional eating, a technique called EFT (Emotional Freedom Technique) or

"Tapping" can be used to help people to release their emotions, instead of stuffing their emotions with food. According to EFT founder Gary Craig, unresolved emotional issues or traumas create blocks or disruptions in the body's subtle energy systems. The energy disruptions create an anxiety short circuit in the body that causes a person to overeat.

EFT is a form of acupuncture, but without needles. You simply tap with your fingertips on a series of acupuncture (or meridian points, which are used in Chinese medicine) on your body while focusing on the emotional food craving. Success is created by releasing the disruption in the body's energy system, instead of having to use willpower to stop the emotional overeating. It has been stated that the success rate of EFT is 70 to 80 percent in the curing of emotional eating.

Some people believe that EFT addresses the energy imbalance in addition to unresolved negative emotions that create the imbalance. EFT is considered to be relaxing, and helps to remove the anxiety that drives emotional eating. It is also believed that the person will eat more nutritionally, because they no longer need to tranquilize their emotions by eating excessive amounts of food.

To release a negative emotion, the EFT technique includes focusing on the negative emotion and saying "even though…" (followed by the negative feelings that you may have) "I completely love and accept myself," while tapping with the fingers on a series of points on the body that relate to certain meridians. (See the following diagrams.) It is believed that the end result is restoring balance to the body's energy field.

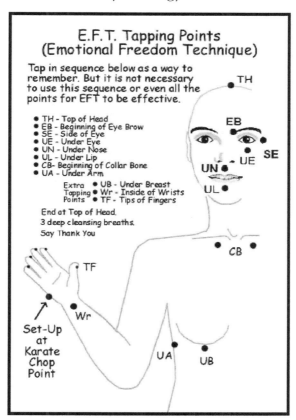

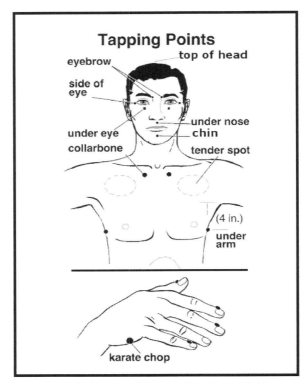

Further information and a free EFT manual can be obtained from: www.emofree.com.

People have also used EFT to help with physical ailments, such as relieving cold symptoms, and the pain from Fibromyalgia. But emotionally, it has helped to ease fear, anxiety, post-traumatic stress disorder, addictions, stress, phobias, grief and feelings of depression. In addition to people achieving emotional peace with EFT, people have used EFT to ease or eliminate their immediate food cravings, and it can help a person to uncover the reason behind their cravings. It is believed that EFT can possibly bring an unresolved emotional memory to the surface so that it can be released. Some people have also said that EFT helped to motivate them to not only start, but continue with an exercise program.

It helps a person's self-esteem, when they are loved and appreciated by their friends who support them. Having someone that you can talk to or communicate with on the web, can be helpful when a person has pent-up emotions that need to be expressed. Releasing the emotions, in addition to being free of the habit of using food to try to balance emotions, is the answer.

Sometimes eating becomes a habit. In which case, it is important to keep in mind that it takes at least three weeks (21 days) to make or break a habit. So, if the person has a habit of eating a particular food each day at a certain time (such as binging on ice cream every evening), it is good to keep in mind that they need to work through releasing that habit for the first few weeks. Try replacing it with some other "reward" that would work for you. Best of all; replace the habit with a healthy habit such as taking a walk, riding a bike or exercise bike, or whatever interests you.

If you think of your body like your car, imagine that if the car stalled, you might have to get out and push it. It can be hard first to get the car to move, but once it gets going, it will feel a lot easier. The same thing can be said for our mind and body. If we can just get through the initial push, it will become easier. And the rewards will come as well, as both you and those around you notice the change.

You can accomplish your goal with the help of a friend, or someone you can talk to while you are going through the experience of trying to release a habit. Maybe that person has a habit he or she is trying to release, and could use your support by having someone with whom to talk as he/she needs to be free from their habit as well.

Your journal can also be an important tool to help you to get through the period of releasing a habit. When you feel like eating, instead of going for food, you can write in the journal about what you are experiencing, and how you feel. You may discover there is an underlying reason for the eating that you did not know existed. Once this reason is brought to the surface, it can be understood and released.

Remember not to be hard on yourself at this time. You are only human, and therefore, have thoughts and emotions. It is important to congratulate yourself for recognizing what is going on, and realizing that you are doing a great job of getting through it as each day passes. And before you know it, you will discover your inner self. Then you will come to understand and appreciate who you really are. After all, there are many things that we endure throughout life, and unless you live in a protective bubble, you are bound to experience many of life's challenges.

Clear Out the Clutter

The weight that you carry in your body may also have to do with the need to hold on to things — the clutter in your life. The clutter that you may have in your house can also be reflected in your body, or the "house" that your soul resides in.

There have been actual cases where people have lost excess weight while organizing, and freeing themselves of excess clutter. Although it may seem difficult to part with something that has a memory attached to it, the result can be helpful for the mind, body and soul.

Un-cluttering your home can be good for emotional and physical reasons. It helps to get rid of dust and germs, and makes it easier to find things. If you are not able to find your athletic shoes, workout items, or sports gear, it is easier to give up and not get the exercise that you need. By clearing out and letting go, it can trigger our mind to let go of our psychological grip on food, and ultimately let go of the grip we have on our weight. Also, by letting go of our focus on food, we can lose the desire to keep eating when we are not hungry.

Whether you have suffered from grief, depression, or some other mental or emotional situation that has led to clutter, it is very healing to let go. Even those people who are hoarders (people who find it impossible and maybe even painful to part with possessions) can be helped with six months of behavioral therapy. The decision to let go of things can trigger the subconscious desire to also release the weight.

How Sleep Affects Us

If we are not able to release and let go of our problems or painful emotions, we can find it difficult to sleep. And getting enough sleep goes back to taking care of ourselves. Researchers at Columbia University studied sleep patterns and obesity rates among participants in the government's National Health and Nutritional Examination Survey. (Seven to nine hours of sleep was considered normal.)

The results of their findings are as follows:

1. Four hours or less of sleep resulted in people being 73% more likely to be obese than those who slept eight hours.

2. Five hours of sleep resulted in people being 50% more likely to be obese.

3. Six hours of sleep resulted in a 23% higher rate of obesity.

The lack of sleep in children has added to the childhood obesity crisis, because of the change in the lifestyles of today's society. And it is not just affecting the children, but everyone. We are not always going to bed when it gets dark, and waking up in the morning light like our ancestors did. We may be staying up late watching television, or working long hours (such as in the case of divorce and a single parent family). The stress alone of the fast-paced world can affect our sleep.

A study by the University of Pennsylvania showed that people who are not getting enough sleep are more likely to choose those fattening magic foods like sweets and high fat foods. When the students had eight hours of sleep, they actually chose healthier foods than when they had four hours of sleep. After only four hours of sleep, they usually chose food for its convenience, rather than preparing it themselves. (See the chapter: Love — The Main Ingredient.)

A lack of sleep and/or too much stress can lead to sleep deprivation and ultimately adrenal fatigue or adrenal exhaustion. This exhaustion signals the body that it is time for some energy, which leads to food cravings. The craving is often sugar or carbohydrate snacks, or too much alcohol. Consuming too much of these foods or alcohol can compound your problem.

Sometimes when we are tired, we are not thinking clearly about what we are eating. We are most likely paying less attention to what we are putting into our mouths. Fatigue causes people to lose their common sense, which affects what they choose to eat. The focus can be on how to stay awake by using high sugar foods when a person is desperate to stay alert while at work or at school. Also, people are most likely not getting the exercise they need when they are tired.

Surprisingly, the university study concluded that sleep deprived people ate *less* food, yet there is an association between a lack of sleep and obesity. (People who do not get enough sleep are more likely to be overweight.) Once again proving that it is not so much about the quantity of food but other factors including the amount of sleep a person is receiving. Researchers at Stanford University also agreed that it is possible to gain weight when a person is eating fewer calories.

Although the belief was that people who gained weight had to be eating more calories, the studies have proven that this is not the case. Another conclusion that has been made is that a loss of sleep slows down the metabolism. In other words, if a person does not get enough sleep and tries to cut back on their eating, they can still gain weight.

Also, it is believed that when a person is tired from a lack of sleep, they may be hungry but have lost their appetite. This is because the loss of sleep also puts stress on the body, triggering a "fight or flight" response. This response is a reaction to alleviate stress. The resulting nervousness can take away a person's appetite.

Not getting the sleep we need, can have a negative affect on the immune system. It can also increase the risk for diabetes and cardiovascular problems. The conclusion is that sleep is just as important as how we eat and whether we exercise. Letting go of what may be troubling us, and getting a good night sleep is important for good health and weight management. Once again, the bottom line is we need to take care of ourselves, and that includes our mind, body and soul.

Another way of letting go and getting the rest that we need is to simply take a vacation. Getting away from it all — going to the ocean or the mountains, or wherever our heart takes us — can really help to give us another perspective on our lives. And sometimes the things that we were holding onto that we thought were so important (but were not beneficial to us) can finally be released. Because after we remove ourselves from the situation, we can often see things more clearly, and the need to hold onto things (or other people) may no longer be there.

Think you cannot afford it? Think again. If there is a will, there is a way, and we can often find that there are other things that we can do without in our lives, so that we are able to put a few dollars away for that much needed trip somewhere. (Not to mention, it can be less expensive than you think if you just open your mind to the possibilities.)

Ultimately, we must love and nurture ourselves in today's hectic world by learning to let go and release, so that we can succeed in managing our weight, and ultimately, keep ourselves healthy. In doing so we not only help ourselves, but it gives us the strength and stamina to help those around us, so that together, we can accomplish anything, including achieving a healthy weight. By connecting with ourselves and letting go, a healthy balance can be found.

10

Re-Connecting with Yourself

Getting my lifelong weight struggle under control has come from a process of treating myself as well as I treat others in every way.

– Oprah Winfrey

When we are children, we can be fearless. It's a time when we can run and play and just enjoy life. As children we have an active imagination. However, we seem to lose touch with this as we become adults. That sense of freedom and imagination could allow us to have fun, enjoy life, and would give us hope to reach our goals. That connection with our inner-child gets lost along the way. This lack of connection can result in using food or other things in excess to help fill the space within us that once felt full and satisfied. But those things can never actually fill that empty space.

There can be times when we have very high expectations for ourselves, which are sometimes based upon what other people want for us. When we do not meet those expectations, the negative emotions can be overwhelming. Binge eating or eating comfort food provides a temporary escape from those emotions, but this discon-nection from self-awareness adversely affects the body. However, if we can learn to love ourselves for who we are and release those high expecta-tions, we can also release the desire to escape from those negative emotions, and ultimately balance our weight.

It is important to love and enjoy our food, but it is even more important to love ourselves. The Bible says, "you shall love your neighbor as yourself." In this day and age, we could also think of it as "love yourself as you can love your neighbor." But people get caught up with their busy lives and they don't pay attention to their own wants and needs. They don't realize that they must re-connect and heal inside. It is then that everything falls into place.

Every now and then, it is a good idea to simply take a moment to re-assess your life. Do you have too much on your plate? This is not just the amount of food that you have, but the amount of things that you've got going on in your life. You can start by prioritizing and making a list.

Are all of the things that take up time in your life actually worthwhile? Sometimes we get involved in things that simply take away time that could be used in a more beneficial way, such as spending time doing things that we enjoy.

Some people who work too hard believe that they are helping their family financially. However, they may actually be working themselves into an early grave. That, of course, doesn't benefit the family. Those material things that people feel they need to provide their family, are probably less meaningful than spending more time with their family.

It is very important to love ones' self. This is a natural state of being — something we are born with. But because of various experiences that effect our lives, that sense of self-esteem can end up being buried away. As a result, there is the disconnection from our true self. That lack of connection to our inner being can lead to filling the emptiness with food — finding comfort in food rather than feeling comfortable with ourselves.

As far as diets go, we need to stop depriving our bodies, and ultimately our inner self. It's time to call a cease fire, and regain our natural balance. By doing so we will find inner peace and contentment with who we are, and our weight can balance out naturally.

Many of the tools that are mentioned in this book come down to one basic concept: Loving and respecting ourselves enough so that we can focus on our own need to find balance in our lives. It's about raising our self-esteem so that we can find the strength to reach whatever goal we wish to achieve, whether the goal is a healthy weight or something else. And above all, to feel connected, so that we do not try to fill the emptiness of feeling disconnected with excessive amounts of food.

In order to feel connected, it is important to be "present" — in the now. Even though your day may be very busy, you can still take a moment to enjoy the sights, sounds and scents of the world around you. Notice the beauty of the sky. Listen to the birds. Look at the beauty of flowers. Or in the winter, the beauty may be in the pure glistening snow.

When you take a break from your job or whatever it is that you do in your daily life, spend some time with yourself. Write in a journal. Enjoy a good book and *feel connected* to the world around you, knowing that everything is connected in some way.

You are part of this big beautiful universe. Think of it like this: The chair that you are sitting on is connected to the ground (or to a building that is connected to the ground), which is connected to the plants, trees, animals, oceans mountains and the entire planet. You are not alone. You are "one" with everything.

Rather than believe that the place in which you dwell and its contents are the only thing that is yours, consider that you are really connected to the whole world. Even if you were "homeless," you would not be homeless because this world is your home. And, it is amazing how many people there are who would be willing to share their home or their belongings with someone else.

Our possessions, and everything in the universe is ever changing. The home that we live in, and other possessions that we "own" are only temporary. But it is our inner being / soul that is eternal. That is the one possession that we can truly call our own. And as a result, we can be our own best friend.

In your daily life, keep in mind that today is the only thing that ever really exists. So don't waste any time, it is important to enjoy the

moment, and the beauty of it is that it doesn't
cost a thing. After all, we are forever evolving,
and once you reach one goal, or obtain another
possession, you will continue to want more. It is
simply human nature.

If we become aware of the constant
connection with ourselves, or our eternal soul,
then no matter what happens around us and no
matter how much things change, we never have
to feel "disconnected." We can feel more
satisfied within ourselves, and have less of a need
to fill the insecure feeling that we may be
experiencing with food.

The 13th century poet and mystic Rumi
understood this when he wrote:

The Journey Starts Here

> Don't go off sightseeing.
> The real journey is right here.
> The great excursion starts from exactly where
>   you are.
> You are the world.
> You have everything you need.
> You are the secret.
> You are the wide opened.
> Don't look for the remedy for your troubles
>   outside yourself.

You are the medicine.
You are the cure for your own sorrow.

Part of loving yourself is treating yourself to things that you enjoy, without using food in excess. What about the little things that make you feel good? For women, it may be getting a massage, manicure or facial. If you can't afford that, then what about a nice hot bath, with some nice relaxing, fragrant bath oil or salt?

For men, it may be getting together with some friends to play cards or sports. Maybe a hike in nature, or going fishing would allow someone to connect with themselves. Sometimes, getting away for the weekend can be a relaxing change. Just think of some way that you can reward yourself, especially when you reach a mile stone in managing your weight. It might simply be a matter of asking yourself: "What do I want to do at this very moment?" Let yourself feel free to have and to do what *you* want at this very moment.

A good question to ask yourself is: Am I doing what I really want to do, or is it what someone else wants me to do? In other words, are you in charge of your destiny? Living your life according to what someone else wants for you is certainly not very inspiring. Figuring out what *you* want is the first step in re-connecting with yourself.

There are certainly goals and dreams that we can create for ourselves. We can use our journal to come up with a list of things we would like to do or accomplish. What could you do that would give you a great sense of joy? Is there something that you have always wanted to try? Is there some goal that would be so fantastic if you accomplished it? Above all, do you feel fulfilled, and if not, are you using food to fill the emptiness? Becoming fulfilled through finding your purpose can release the need to fill yourself with food. And when you consider your options in life, just keep in mind that anything is possible.

If you think you haven't got what it takes, think again. Give yourself a chance, and above all, be patient. When we accomplish those dreams and goals, we can begin to feel better about ourselves. And often, all it takes is determination and persistence. The goal can be anything, and while we become busy and absorbed in our own accomplishments, we can become less focused on food. When we take our mind off of food, we stop thinking about not eating.

Sometimes when people have achieved a healthy weight, they reward themselves by taking a dream vacation. But even before that, they choose to reward themselves (sometimes with special meals) at each milestone (such as a change in clothing size). And when a person's soul is filled with the joys and rewards of life, then they no longer crave the things that will never fill it, such as excess food.

How people view themselves in society can affect their weight. A study of teenage girls revealed that where a girl sees herself on the social ladder affects how much her weight will increase. As part of the study, the following question was asked: "At the top of the ladder, are the people in your school with the most respect and the highest standing; at the bottom are the people who no one respects and no one wants to hang around with; where do you place yourself on the ladder?"

The girls were then split into two groups: The girls who said they were at rung five or above, and the girls who said they were on rung four or below. Those girls who thought they were unpopular gained more weight during a two year period than girls who thought they were popular. The average age of the girls was 15, and they all gained *some* weight. But the girls who rated themselves very low in popularity were 69 percent more likely to gain about 11 pounds. The girls who ranked themselves more highly on the popularity scale gained some weight, but the weight gain averaged 6½ pounds.

And, it did not matter what race or household income the girl was from. The results were the same. Above all, their view of themselves, or their level of self-esteem, could actually affect their health. Ultimately, it was determined that how a teenage girl feels about herself should be part of the strategy to prevent adolescent obesity. It became apparent that when adults set high standards in the schools, students actually treat each other with more respect.

Having a healthy self-esteem is important at any age, and improving our self-esteem is another important weight-management tool. Sometimes we enter a career that we are not passionate about, but we do it because someone told us to, or we believed that it was the "right" thing to do. We may have found ourselves in a situation with a tough decision to make, and went in a direction that did not fit who we truly are.

The inner peace that we felt as a child was replaced by duty. With each step that we took in life, we continued to believe that our wants and needs were not important, as we completely lost our connection with ourselves.

Although we thought that we were doing the right thing by perhaps putting other people's wants and needs above our own, we were not actually helping them. Eventually there came a time when we no longer functioned at our optimum level. Instead we buried ourselves in food, or deprived ourselves by dieting to try and gain some control.

Hopefully we can realize that we are not helping ourselves, and understand we are not really helping others. It's like when on an airplane, and the flight attendant instructs us that in case of a change in cabin pressure, the oxygen masks will drop, and we are told to make sure that we give ourselves oxygen first before we help others with their oxygen.

If you apply that to your life, you may at first believe that it is selfish. But we must respect ourselves, before we can truly help others. If we do not nurture our soul, our ability to nurture others becomes eroded. So our loss of our connection with our sense of self becomes a loss of a connection with others, and in a sense, our connection with God.

Some people go from one bad relationship to another in order to avoid being alone. But, if they would only give themselves time to get used to being on their own, they would make the best connection in their life. By developing our love of self, we can then finally attract the person who is right for us. And that person will most likely be someone that will allow us to be ourselves. In the end, our connection to our self results in a meaningful connection with other people.

Usually, if we are doing what we enjoy, we find ourselves around other people with similar interests. Those similarities help our connection with other people, and can form lasting friendships. Those friendships can provide much needed support. When it comes to weight management, support can be very powerful. This concept can be used to help us achieve success in other areas of our lives.

Through re-connecting with ourselves and others, we can discover our true purpose. By doing the things that we are meant to do in our life, we can feel a greater sense of satisfaction. It feeds our soul in a way that food cannot. And, if we try to use food to fill that emptiness, we will never feel satisfied.

Sometimes we become desperate to find the answers "out there." We buy diet book after diet book, and search endlessly for the answer to our weight imbalance. But, the answers are really *on the inside*, and may have to do with a person's identity. For example, a woman begins her life as someone's daughter. Then they become a girl-friend, a wife, and a mother, and then they may wonder who they really are. After all, besides understanding her body, a woman also needs to connect with the essence of her true self.

This identity goes beyond being a woman, beyond family expectations, and beyond hormone fluctuations. This process of self-discovery includes removing false layers of identity, going back through all of the person's beliefs, and realizing what they are *not*. During the self-discovery process a person should start asking themselves some questions.

The most important question can be: "Who am I really?" It is not your name, address, or social security number. And, certainly not the number on a bathroom scale. But who are you really on the inside? What are you passionate about? Was that passion suppressed by some sense of responsibility? What were your dreams as a child? What would you like to do with your life that makes you feel passionate? Try writing it down (no matter what other people may think). Is there any way that you could pursue that dream? Just open your mind to the possibilities. It's never too late. Many people who become highly successful in their careers, are often past the age of 50. Look at the successful business people out there, and some of them are still going, even though they are long past "retirement" age.

A tool that people have used to help them to connect with their inner self through awareness, and to understand who they truly are, is meditation. (See the chapter called: Breathe.) Meditation does not cost anything, and it does not require professional training. It is simply something that can be done on your own, and has many benefits, including helping you to find answers to questions that you may have.

Women have even found meditation to be useful when they are pregnant. Daily meditation can become a precious time to make sense of the many thoughts and feelings that can be running through the mind of a mother-to-be. It can help her to connect with her emotions, and reduce any feeling of stress that she may be experiencing. This can also reduce the need for emotional eating, and excessive weight gain during pregnancy.

Finding Balance

In order to find balance in our weight, it can help to find balance in the basic areas of our lives. Do you feel completely satisfied in all areas of your life? To find out, create the following chart and circle the number next to the area of your life that represents your level of satisfaction. Number one represents no satisfaction, and number ten is completely satisfied.

AREA	LOW SATISFACTION					HIGH SATISFACTION				
Family:	1	2	3	4	5	6	7	8	9	10
Friends:	1	2	3	4	5	6	7	8	9	10
Romance:	1	2	3	4	5	6	7	8	9	10
Finances/Money:	1	2	3	4	5	6	7	8	9	10
Health:	1	2	3	4	5	6	7	8	9	10
Living Area:	1	2	3	4	5	6	7	8	9	10
Fun & Recreation:	1	2	3	4	5	6	7	8	9	10
Career:	1	2	3	4	5	6	7	8	9	10
Spiritual:	1	2	3	4	5	6	7	8	9	10

After you have finished circling one number for each area, you can take a look at how satisfied you are in the basic areas of your life. This helps to give you focus, so that you know where to begin. It is helpful to focus on one area at a time because if you go in too many directions at once, it can make it more difficult to achieve your goals.

Start with the area that has the lowest number, and ask yourself: What would make that area of my life a ten? For example, if the lowest number is three and it is in the area of Friends, then take a moment to imagine what you would really like to have in that area. If it is more friends that you would like to have, then how could you go about connecting with people in order to make more friends? Or maybe there is a particular person that you would like to meet or get to know.

Once you have determined what you want in order to improve that area of your life, you can use various tools that are mentioned in this book. You can use your imagination to visualize how you wish to be, you can write an affirmation and put it somewhere where you will see it every day, you can create a vision board with pictures and words that describe how you want to be, you can use self-hypnosis or write in your journal, among other things.

By using some of the tools along with taking steps toward improving that area, you can get closer to being fully satisfied in that area. When you feel you are satisfied in that area, then you can move on to the area with the next lowest number. In summary, when we find balance in our lives it will ultimately balance our weight, because we no longer need to try to satisfy ourselves with food.

Meeting our Needs

Loving ourselves includes understanding our own needs. And you may have needs in your life that are not being met. Those needs may seem simple to you. But getting in touch with those needs can be very important in order to connect with your self. Below are some important questions that you can ask yourself. If the answers to these questions are "no," then how can you fulfill those needs?

Copy this page onto a sheet of paper, and then try answering the following questions.

1. Do you feel accepted? Yes No

2. Do you feel that you are growing and learning? Yes No

3. Do you feel healthy? Yes No

4. Do you feel safe and secure? Yes No

5. Do you have enough freedom? Yes No

6. Do you feel respected? Yes No

7. Do you feel that you are enjoying your life? Yes No

8. Do you feel loved? Yes No

9. Do you feel supported? Yes No

10. Are you fulfilling your need to be creative? Yes No

If you answered no to any of these questions, take your time to think about what you would like to receive in your life, so that you can feel that the need is being met. Simply copy the following and fill in the blank next to each answer that you said no to.

I will feel accepted by _____

I will grow and learn by _____

I will feel healthier by _____

I will feel safe and secure by _____

I will feel free by _____

I will feel respected by _____

I will enjoy life more by _____

I will feel loved by _____

I will feel supported by _____

I will feel more creative by _____

You can then allow these desires to come into your life by creating an affirmation. An affirmation helps us to receive our desires by focusing on the things that we want and need in our life in a *positive* way. It uses the power of the subconscious mind, which responds to positive suggestion.

It is at the subconscious level that we can more easily make the changes that we desire to make. Otherwise, our thoughts can be rejected at the conscious level. It is important to *feel positive* when saying or thinking about the affirmation. That positive feeling can clear away the negative thoughts that stop us from receiving what we need, and allows us to make the positive change in our lives. Another way to clear away any negative thoughts is to feel some appreciation. By using appreciation, we can completely change the way we feel, which opens our mind to receive the suggestion.

You can create your affirmation by filling in the blanks (with examples in parenthesis).

Your affirmation:

I feel appreciative that

_____ (ie: I am learning)

now that I am _____

(reaching my goal).

If you wish to simply focus on your weight, you could also say something like:

"I am so appreciative, now that I am <u>healthy</u>, <u>happy</u> and <u>at my ideal weight</u>."

Or, fill in the blanks:

I am so appreciative, now that I am _____

_____, _____,

and _____.

It is good to remember to not use more than three desires at a time. And, try to use the same affirmation for as long as possible without giving up on your desire. You will also notice that the affirmation is in the present tense. For example, if we tell ourselves that we *will* have it, then our subconscious mind believes that it will happen sometime in the future. And as the saying goes, tomorrow may never come. In our mind, there is only today. So remember to be positive, be present, and be patient. Faith is also important.

After you have your affirmation, you can read it out loud to yourself twice each day (in the morning and in the evening before bed), and imagine and *believe* that you already have what you desire. You must also *feel* the positive emotion along with the affirmation in order for it to be effective. It is a good idea to say it at bedtime, because it helps the thought to sink into the subconscious mind as you sleep. You can also write the affirmation on a post-it note, and put it somewhere where you will see it each day. (For example: in your car, or on the bathroom mirror.)

A good exercise for maintaining a positive mental attitude, especially for those people who like to journal, is to keep an appreciation journal. It can be especially helpful to keep it near the bed, and write in it at bedtime. You can simply write down a few things that you appreciate. It is also a good idea to be as specific as possible. For example, you may appreciate your children. But now say exactly what it is about them that you appreciate.

You will find that no matter how difficult life becomes, and no matter what "bad" things occur in your life, there is always something to appreciate. And if nothing else, we can just appreciate life.

No matter who we are, or whatever goal we are trying to achieve, it is important to remain optimistic and to believe that we can achieve whatever we can imagine. A good reminder of this is the following saying, which came from President Calvin Coolidge.

Press On

Nothing in this world can take the place of persistence.

Talent will not; nothing is more common than unsuccessful people with talent.

Genius will not; unrewarded genius is almost a proverb.

Education will not; the world is full of educated derelicts.

Persistence and determination alone are omnipotent.

Ultimately, the answer to feeling fulfilled is not in being "filled" with food. If you simply allow yourself to re-connect with who you really are, and believe that you are loved, you can begin to feel satisfied; mentally, emotionally and physically. Besides, we must love ourselves in order to have self-preservation, and to truly allow ourselves to be respected by others. And when you make that transformation, you may be surprised at what (or who) you have found.

11

Connecting with Others

This is why I loved the support groups so much. If people thought you were dying, they gave you their full attention. If this might be the last time they saw you, they really saw you. People listened instead of just waiting for their turn to speak. And when they spoke, they weren't telling you a story. When the two of you talked, you were building something, and afterward you were both different than before.

– Chuck Palahniuk, *Fight Club*

*Y*ou've heard this before: "The number you are trying to reach has been temporarily disconnected." This can also be said of the way we feel at times. When we come into this world, there is an inherent physical "disconnect" from our mother as the cord is cut, and if you are so inclined to believe — our connection with the serene world that we left behind. This could leave us with a perpetual longing for the loving connection we once experienced.

As we go through life, many relationships come to an end. This can include family, friends and romantic relationships. When we graduate from a class, we may feel that we have disconnected from the friends that we had become so close to. And this can happen more than once as we go from grade school to high school, and perhaps on to college. When we leave home, we may feel that we have lost the close connection that we had with our parents. Or maybe our parents got divorced, and we felt some resentment over what we felt was a lost connection to one of our parents.

Perhaps we went through a divorce, or simply ended a boy/girl relationship, which generally happens several times in our lives. And then there is the ultimate loss, when somebody close to us passes away, again leaving us with a feeling of a loss of connection. No matter how we may hope and wish that we could talk to them or see them one more time, we can be left with a hopeless sense of despair and loss.

Sometimes we have to move because of our job, or for some other reason, removing us from our familiar surroundings and neighbors with whom we may have formed a bond. All of these things, and many more occurrences that naturally happen in this life of ours can leave us feeling isolated, and we may feel as though we are all alone in this world.

Although we may feel completely alone at times, we really are not, because in fact, we are all connected. We just can't see it, but, we can find a way to *feel* it. We may appear to be different from the outside, but in reality, we all come from the same source. We are all here in this world to learn, and to experience life. It is like being at school, and although we come from different backgrounds, races, religions, nationalities, etc., we all have similar hopes, dreams, fears and insecurities.

People who feel financially poor, may look at those people who have more money and material possessions, and feel disconnected from them. But what they don't see, is what is *really* going on in those people's lives. If they knew the reality of the other person's pain or challenges, their envy or feeling of disconnection might actually turn to pity, and the "poor" people might actually realize how blessed they truly are.

This is why people will pay a lot of money for candid pictures of the rich and famous going through difficult times. It can make us realize that they are no different than anyone else, and that having money does not guarantee happiness.

There was a woman who was wearing a six carat diamond ring, and another woman that was sitting next to her commented on the beautiful ring. But the woman with the big diamond ring said, "I would gladly trade it for good health." She was having health issues that all of the money in the world could not fix.

Money only goes so far, and the rich and famous people suffer as anyone else does, but perhaps in different ways. Also, for some people it will never be enough, and they can never be satisfied, no matter how much money they have. This is because true happiness comes from *within* us. It cannot be bought. Happiness and appreciation need to come first, before one can experience prosperity. Often the best things in life are free, like having the love of family and friends who help us to feel connected.

Is food your best friend? If so, maybe its time to make some new friends. And when you do, the weight can simply "melt" away. That's what happened to Nancy Makin. Nancy had reached 703 pounds after spending many years living alone in her one bedroom apartment. She estimated that she left the house only eight times in 12 years.

During that time, she continued to bury her feelings in food. Her son would bring her 10 double cheeseburgers. She would eat four of them, and put the rest in the refrigerator. Later, sometimes during the night, she would eat them cold, or she would eat anything else that was available.

She ate to try to make herself feel better from the loneliness and boredom she experienced after her divorce. But the use of food to make her feel better never lasted very long. As Nancy said, "You are stuffing your feelings... substituting the real thing that will make you feel whole for food, and food does not last." During that time, Nancy only allowed her family to see her, and would send her son to get her groceries.

At one point, Nancy's sister gave her a computer, and she began reaching out to people. She created an entire social life on the computer. As Nancy stated, "I wasn't trying to lose weight, I was just reaching out." The friends that she made online did not judge her by how she looked. After all, they could not see her. Instead, they loved and appreciated Nancy for who she was on the *inside*. Nancy wrote, "the anonymity of the computer gave me access to a world that would have just as well have left me alone, alone to die, but I did not."

Often times Nancy simply discussed politics, but the friends that she made, gave her a sense of value in herself, and she became happier. She said, "I was being loved and nurtured by faceless strangers, and friends accepted who I was based on my mind and soul." People thought that Nancy was smart and funny, and those friendships helped her to connect with her true self. She said: "It was anonymous. I didn't have that barrier there. They saw my wit, and they saw my intelligence, and I was not in that shell."

With all of the connecting that Nancy accomplished on the computer (up to 12 to 13 hours per day), she had less time to think about eating. She stopped consuming those large amounts of food, and as she did, the weight began to disappear. Nancy did not watch the scale. She did not count calories, or take any diet pills. She did not cut entire food groups (such as carbohydrates) out of her diet, or eat any special pre-packaged food. She simply was too busy connecting with people, and by doing so, she connected with herself.

Nancy said, "I never knew how much I was losing because it didn't matter. That is the key. It didn't matter." The entire process brought her to some important realizations. As Nancy said, "I've heard so many times, I said it myself, if I could only lose 40 or 50 pounds, I'd be so much happier. I've found on this journey that the opposite is true." After her weight dropped by 400 pounds, she began to go out in public again, and seeing people face to face. She developed confidence in herself, and that confidence is so important in reaching any goal, whether it is weight, career, or anything else.

Since losing a total of 530 pounds, Nancy was invited on the Oprah Winfrey show. She has also been invited on to other programs, as she shares her story with the hope that she can empower other people to help themselves. As ABC News reported, Nancy got her weight down to "a healthy 170 pounds." After her loneliness and isolation, she is now inspired to speak to people and create the connection that she found, which allowed her to appreciate herself for the beautiful person that she is.

Although, nowadays, in our fast-paced society we get caught up in connecting with people through email, voice mail and text messaging, it is better to take it a step further and meet with people one-on-one or in a group. If at first you do not feel confident enough, then a relationship can be built through "cyber space" and then you may feel comfortable enough to get to know someone in person.

The Importance of "Touch"

With all of the stress we may be feeling in our lives, and all of the decisions that we have to make, we can become disconnected from our body and our energy level can drop since our energy is mostly going to our head instead. As a result, our ability to sleep can be negatively affected. But being physically touched by someone can regain that mind-body connection and actually improve our ability to regain our energy.

After all, there is definitely a healing power in human touch. In fact, being touched can help a person's immune system to become stronger by increasing the amount of white blood cells in a person's body. Touching can also decrease anxiety. Touching can slow down the heart rate, and decrease blood pressure. From an emotional standpoint, it can increase the endorphin levels in the brain which makes you feel good. The more touching you receive, the better it is for you.

Our skin is the largest organ in the human body, with about 8,000 receptors in an area the size of a finger tip. When the skin is touched, our nerve fibers send messages to the spinal chord, and on to the brain. People who are in a coma may respond to the feeling of touch as someone holds their hand, which can change their heart rate. Touching someone can release endorphins, which help to suppress pain.

Touching is really necessary for a person to live a healthy life. Getting a massage can be very beneficial for stress relief and for boosting the immune system. In some people, massage has made a positive impact on conditions such as diabetes, migraines and asthma. Instead of using comfort food to feel better, try getting some comfort from soothing touch.

A woman's skin is actually more sensitive to touch than a man's skin. Her stress level can be high because she has less of the chemicals that help to relieve stress. Because of this, a woman can more benefit from and appreciate the healing power of touch. If a woman feels that people are not reaching out to her, she can "break the ice" by touching.

A person can begin by giving someone a hug, or they can kiss a friend on the cheek if they feel like it.

Hugging helps to de-stress us by giving us that warm sense of connection with another human being. You may be surprised with the pleasant reaction from the other person. If you don't want to hug, you can try giving someone a re-assuring pat on the back. If it is someone that you feel close enough to, you could walk arm in arm with them.

It can also make someone feel good if you touch their hand when you are talking with them, and when you make someone else feel good, it can make you feel good as well. Giving massages can be even more beneficial than receiving them. It can help to reduce a sense of loneliness and depression. Doctor visits can become fewer, and people become more sociable when they experience physical contact with someone.

It's like the old saying "what goes around, comes around." In a study it was found that when waitresses touched their customers (either on the shoulder or on the hand) when they gave change back, they actually received a larger tip.

People have a tendency to remember when a person was kind to them, especially in times of stress or sorrow. Then when you need a "hand to hold," that person is more likely to be there for you. Therefore, why not just make a difference in someone's life with a little touch?

Touching premature babies can be a matter of life or death. It has been shown that babies actually require human touch. Without it, they do not grow normally. The Touch Research Institute (TRI) at the University of Miami is a leading scientific center that explores how touch affects health. TRI studies premature babies and how their development is affected by touch by giving them gentle massages each day while they are in their incubator.

They discovered that giving the premature babies massages for ten days helps them to be more alert, responsive and active than babies that were not massaged, and they gain weight 47 percent faster. (It has also helped to ease colic.) Premature babies that were massaged were discharged from the hospital an average of six days sooner than babies who were not.

If a child is not touched often enough, they can grow up to be physically violent. In addition, massage has helped autistic children with their ability to concentrate. To provide touch to your children, you can snuggle with them when you watch television, or rub their back when they are sleeping. Children can feel more secure and loved at a young age when they crawl into their parent's bed at night.

In this fast-paced stress-filled society, people are getting more massages than ever, which may be because they are not receiving enough physical touch in their daily lives. With the growing concern that society has over sexual harassment and child abuse, the concern is that American's are not receiving enough human touch. In fact, when couples were studied at cafes in various countries, it was determined that the highest rate of touch was in Puerto Rico, and the U.S. was in the lower range of the study group. As a result, this lack of touch can negatively affect an individual's growth and emotional wellbeing.

Because touching in the workplace can make people feel uncomfortable, it should be done in a friendship or family situation where it is considered acceptable. And of course we should not be touching certain areas of the body, such as the chest, buttocks or below the belt, especially when it comes to children. A man may feel more uncomfortable about hugging than a woman, so you can first try to give them a tap on the shoulder instead.

Couples can find not only stress relief, but an added connection to each other when they rub each other's back, shoulders, neck or feet. A foot massage or foot reflexology helps your energy to move from your head into your body. There are many acupuncture points in the feet, which can help to heal other areas of the body.

Getting in the habit of giving and receiving touch can be a warm, healing experience. When it comes to achieving a healthy weight, touching others and being touched can provide the comfort and connection that we crave.

Providing Support

When it comes to connecting with others, it is our friends and those family members that love us unconditionally that can provide the support that we need to reach whatever goal we are trying to attain. They can help us by simply listening as we release our pain, and ultimately release the excess weight that we have been holding on to.

For those people who do not have a family (or a family that is able to provide support), a person can still connect with people that can provide the support they crave. When people open themselves to others they are able to begin to gain support from them. Although they may not have parents, children, or brothers and sisters of their own, they can create relationships that are just as close with people who are like a mother, father, son, daughter, brother or sister.

And in some ways it may be an even better relationship than they had, or could have had with someone that they were biologically connected to, because they can *choose* to have these people in their life. In doing so, they can fill their world with all the love and support they need, by creating that connection. They can also find some unconditional love in a pet, which can help to ease whatever loneliness and isolation that they may be experiencing.

A study was conducted at George Washington University Medical Center with women who had been diagnosed with early breast cancer. It was discovered that the women who had many friends and relatives, whom they could connect with, had a 60 percent lower rate of cancer death or recurrence during a seven year period.

The women who had only two or less people outside the home, whom they could rely on for support, had a 60 percent higher rate of returning breast cancer that was fatal. In other words, the amount of friends that a woman has can actually improve her cancer survival rate. Not only that, but married cancer patients have generally survived longer that unmarried cancer patients.

Another study by Dr. David Spiegel of Stanford University School of Medicine found that breast cancer patients that were involved in support groups lived almost twice as long as the women who were at the same illness level but were not involved in support groups. Dr. Spiegel's research showed that expressing emotions and connecting with people regarding the difficult subject of cancer enhances a person's quality of life, and can increase the life expectancy of people with terminal illnesses.

Although an article by sociologist James House indicated that isolation is bad for a person's health, his study concluded that marriage helps men, but women help other women whether married or not. In other words, women seem to be more help to each other than men, and they make up 70-80 percent of the people who are in Wellness Community groups, which are for cancer patients along with their loved ones. This may be because men often do not talk about their problems and fears. Actually, men need support as much as women. They just don't require as large a group, and they may express themselves in different ways.

A UCLA study confirmed the healing power of friendships among women. The study was called "Female Responses to Stress: Tend and Befriend, Not Fight or Flight." The study showed that by gathering with friends in a way that is nurturing, helps women to lower stress. Women's brains actually release chemicals such as oxytocin that give them the desire to gather with other women, in addition to tending to children. And the more time that a woman spends with friends, the more they release oxytocin.

The friendship that women have with other women helps them to connect with the power of their feminine spirit in a way that enhances their life. Some women's groups refer to themselves as a gathering of "Goddesses." This gives the women an added sense of self-esteem, making them feel beautiful and powerful, and giving them the ability to empower each other to grow. This can create an overall sense of well-being, not to mention a spiritual inspiration when a person feels that someone else believes in them.

A report that was released by Eric Loucks, an instructor at Harvard School of Public Health indicated that having family and close friends is actually good for a person's heart. In addition, it was discovered that connections to religious groups, a community, or having a partner that a person feels close to can also help. The heart study found that men who are socially isolated had increased levels of a blood marker for inflammation. The blood marker has been associated with cardiovascular disease.

Support groups, or "psychosocial inter-ventions," have done a great deal to enhance the quality of life for people who are suffering from a wide range of illnesses. It allows them to not have to face the illness on their own. The group concept has been used with HIV patients, especially to help relieve the stress and grief that they may have experienced by being exposed to the illness. This meaningful support has provided encouragement for patients to express their emotions. When it comes to longevity and support, a study actually showed that mortality rates are higher during the first year after a spouse dies, because the person has lost the support they received from their spouse on a day-to-day basis.

People who are in support groups bond with each other. The group also gives a person a sense of acceptance, and they feel as though they belong. It gives them a chance to share a common dilemma, which can make a person feel less isolated, and it gives them a social network. Also, the group helps people to develop new coping strategies for their situation.

When it comes to weight, groups such as Weight Watchers have had success by providing much needed support. Also, many women have experienced weight management success at Curves, which is a women's-only exercise facility where women can connect with each other as they work out.

Other than the support groups, some additional tips for connecting with people include: Bonding with your family and accepting their "quirks," try to get along with your in-laws and neighbors and learning to compromise. If you find it difficult to get along with someone, it can help to make a list of the positive aspects of that person.

If you can reach out and help others, you can begin to feel the connection. Helping people through volunteering, or some other service, can take your mind off of your own issues, and make you realize that you are not alone. (And your own problems may appear small compared to others.) When you are no longer focused on your problems, then those problems can lose the intensity that they once had.

When we realize that we are all connected, then there is no longer a need to feel that we are alone. Finding a sense of connection with others can help to take our minds off of food. If the focus is removed, we can take away the reason to try and satisfy our problems with food. We can become satisfied through our service or connection to others, and the emptiness inside can be filled. Permanent weight loss (or weight gain, if needed) can then occur.

Of course, there is a difference between being a humanitarian and being a martyr. We should always take care of ourselves, and treat ourselves with respect. Maintaining a healthy sense of self-esteem is crucial to balancing our weight. (See the chapter: Re-Connecting with Yourself.) At the same time, learning to help those who are receptive to our help, and who appreciate the assistance that we can give them, can give us a sense of satisfaction like no other.

The concept of having support has been in existence for a long time. In the book "Think and Grow Rich," Napoleon Hill talks about a "mastermind group." Mr. Hill states that a mastermind is a "coordination of knowledge and effort, in a spirit of harmony, between two or more people, for the attainment of a definite purpose." He states that "no individual may have greater power without availing himself of the Master Mind."

Our ideas as individuals can be like pieces to a puzzle, and when we come together as a group, it is like putting the pieces to the puzzle together to solve a problem. The collective wisdom of the group can help to propel each of us toward our goal, whether the goal is to achieve and maintain a healthy weight, or some other purpose.

More recent books have been written that are aimed at organizations, in order tap into the power of the group. One such book is called: "The Wisdom of Crowds — why the many are smarter than the few and how collective wisdom shapes business, economies, societies and nations." The book discusses how the combined intelligence that is contained within organizations can result in superior decisions. Those decisions are often better than the decisions that a person can make on their own.

In the business world, the power of connecting or networking with other business people is a very valuable tool. Business owners often discover the power of connecting in order to build their business, and gain referrals. Referrals are important because advertising is everywhere in our society, and people often become "de-sensitized" to it. They become so used to seeing or hearing ads all of the time (whether it is on radio, television, on the internet, in magazines or newspapers), that they do not even pay attention to it anymore.

As a result, people often prefer to get a referral from someone they know, before they purchase a particular product or service. They feel that they can trust the advice of a friend or relative that has already had experience with the product or service, rather than believing an ad that a company has simply paid for. This is why some of the best advertising is done through referrals and connecting with people to help sell their product or service.

When we connect with others, such as in support groups, we can come across other people who have been in similar circumstances, such as in the case of grief, and they can provide support and advice on how they were able to overcome their situation. And when we connect and resolve the issue, it can allow us to achieve a healthy weight.

For example, in a support group situation, someone might begin to discuss the pain from Fibromyalgia and how the doctor treated them as if it was "all in their head." The stress from the pain, in addition to being treated as if it was imaginary, resulted in weight gain. Maybe the person found comfort in food, and also had difficulty getting some exercise because of their physical pain.

Someone in the group might mention a similar experience, and then discuss how they managed to get through it and what they did that was helpful. The benefit of this is that we cannot truly know what it is like to live through something unless we have actually "been there." This sense of rapport between two or more people can bring relief to someone who felt alone and "disconnected." This new connection can bring a sense of connection with ourselves, knowing that we are not alone in this world, and that there are other people who are experiencing the same things.

When this is realized there is a feeling of comfort, and the "comfort food" can no longer be needed. Also, they may have new information, or "tools" provided by the other person to help them find relief from their pain, both physically and emotionally.

When we gather people together, instead of having the experience of just ourselves we now may have hundreds of years of life experience. That experience is a wealth of knowledge that can be drawn from. It's like an instant encyclopedia of wisdom from living, along with the combined understanding from the level of the soul's experience. In other words, "support can be beautiful."

In the end, the power of the group can help to propel you more quickly toward your goal, with the combined knowledge, support and connection of a group of people. Simply connecting with others in your daily life also leads to a longer, happier and healthier life. Your worries will become fewer, and therefore the emotional eating can be decreased, or it can disappear completely. Your sense of well-being will be greater, and you will live a more satisfying and joy-filled life.

12

The Ultimate Connection

*The church is within yourself and not in any pope
nor preacher, nor in any building but in self! For
thy body is indeed the temple of the living God.*
— **Edgar Cayce**

*T*he ultimate connection involves connecting with our higher self, and also God. When we think of God, we may think of a church, or a temple. But we can have that divine connection anywhere, twenty-four hours a day, seven days a week. We can tap into that connection to fill the emptiness that we may have felt from the time that we were born, or from any of life's experiences that has made us feel empty. And the creative means that we may use to create that connection, can leave us with a sense of satisfaction and nourishment.

213

In the case of weight, we may be searching for the answer through food, but the answer never comes. The comfort and unconditional love that we seek is never actually satisfied by over-eating, and over-filling ourselves with too much rich food. The concept of a diet can leave us feeling even more deprived than when we began the diet.

You may believe in the divine, or if not, you can simply look at the scientific concept of energy. We know that energy exists, and that it moves through objects (including ourselves) at all times. Using that energy to our benefit, can assist us in healing ourselves both physically and emotionally. And as we use the energy, it is important to focus on the positive, and to imagine that we are *already* the way that we wish to be in addition to feeling grateful for it.

When we are searching for inspiration, there are various divine sources that can provide the inspiration that we need to succeed to reach our goals. This inspiration can give us the added strength of a connection to our source. That inspiration can simply come from the words of others, such as people like Rumi.

Rumi (Mawlana Jalal-ad-Din Muhammad Rumi) was a mystic who lived in the area of

Turkey in the 13th century. A mystic can be described as someone who believes in the existence of realities beyond human comprehension. Rumi was a poet who felt empathy toward people, animals and plants.

Rumi understood the importance of feeling connected to God, and his writings have helped people to connect with the Divine for many centuries. His popularity in the west has grown in recent years, with people feeling inspired by his deep love of the Divine. The following poem by Rumi speaks to the modern-day issue of weight management.

The Best Nourishment

Life on earth has its ups and downs.
Sometimes it's pleasant; sometimes not.
You'd better fall in love with someone who will
*   make you the immortal sultan.*

Since everyone's life is black and white,
Search another life
Made from the radiance of God's light.

O one who has gotten lost in himself,
You're not aware that your life has become a
*   grave.*
In fact, you are buried in the grave of yourself.

Finding the one who gave you life
Is the best nourishment for you.
Yet you are running like fire from one store
To the other
For the food than can be measured
In cups.

That poem was written almost 800 years ago, and has withstood the test of time. Even though it is ancient, the message is still the same. Again, we are talking about the loss of connection to the Divine. This sense of loss can feel like grief to those people who have an insatiable craving to fill the emptiness. We can try to comfort ourselves with food, but food never completely fills the emptiness.

The following excerpt is from the Rumi poem *Song of the Reed*:

Since I was cut from the reedbed,
I have made this crying sound.
Anyone apart from someone he loves
understands what I say.
Anyone pulled from a source longs to go back.

In this poem the word "source" or the "reedbed" refers to God and paradise. It refers to man's life on earth, and his or her quest to return to the Divine. It is believed that the Mathnawi (Rumi's six-volume masterpiece) had one single purpose: Communion with God.

Rumi's work can help fill the need in today's society to find joy in our daily living. Current fans of Rumi's writing have found comfort in his poems during difficult times. In a similar way, Rumi triumphed over trying circumstances of his day. It has been suggested that Rumi's strength and his belief in the Divine, resulted from the difficulties that he experienced in his childhood.

Simply reading his poetry can provide encouragement and inspiration, knowing that some things never change. And no matter what century it is, we carry the common thread of trying to fulfill ourselves with a sense of meaning, purpose and love. But the sense of love has never really left us, because it is *inside* of us, rather than being *out there* somewhere, as in the case of food.

In our search for love through food, we often do not realize that there is instant unconditional love, if we allow ourselves to feel it. Try putting a smile on your face, sense the love in your heart, and believe that you are continually supported, even though you may not *see* it. By tapping into that *feeling*, we can fill the emptiness that we sometimes try to fill with food. And by releasing our troubles to God or our higher self, we can take the weight off of our own shoulders.

The Power of Prayer

By tapping into our heart, we can enter into our soul, and connect with our higher power. As I stated before, there are various tools that can assist us to make the connection. One of these is prayer, which can help us to feel a connection to the Divine. Prayer also allows us to get in touch with our emotions, so that we can connect with our feelings rather than stuffing them with food. Sometimes praying leads to tears, which provides a release from emotional pain that we may have been holding on to.

Some people use the Serenity Prayer for weight management. The Serenity Prayer is also used in 12-step programs. *God grant me the serenity to accept the things I cannot change; the courage to change the things I can; and the wisdom to know the difference.*

The Serenity Prayer helps us to let go of all of the things that we cannot control in life. It reminds us to realize that we need to release our tension and worries. Especially when one spends time worrying about something we have no control over. That time can be better spent empowering ourselves to make the changes that we are able to make, in order to feel more connected to ourselves, and ultimately to God.

Overeaters Anonymous is a twelve step program. Those twelve steps include the statement that "we admitted we were powerless over food — that our lives had become unmanageable," and that we "came to believe that a power greater than ourselves could restore us to sanity." The eleventh step states that we "sought through prayer and meditation to improve our conscious contact with God *as we understood Him*, praying only for knowledge of His will for us and the power to carry that out."

We have the ability to heal ourselves. Just like our body can heal itself, we are able to heal our emotions. Whether it is through daily affirmations (which is like praying), meditating or using visualization, we can connect with our higher self to imagine and feel that we are well. Or in the case of weight management, seeing ourselves happy, and at a healthy weight.

And when you pray, rather than just saying the words (sometimes repeatedly), it is important to mean what you say. In order to help you do that, you can create your own prayer. Also, there are books that contain prayers specifically for weight problems. But personalizing a prayer can be beneficial in creating the right words that fit your situation. You can use your journal to practice writing your prayers. Try starting with the words: Dear God, or whatever introduction works for you.

You can create a prayer each day, or you can create a prayer on the weekend that can be read each day of the week. (A prayer then becomes like an affirmation.) That prayer may even fit whatever situation that you may be going through at that time. The prayer does not have to be specifically for weight, since there is often an underlying issue behind a person's emotional eating. The following is an example of a prayer for weight management:

> *Dear God*
> *As I walk along the path of life,*
> *Help me to find the way to a healthy weight.*
> *As I search for the answer to health and*
>   *well-being,*
> *I ask you to empower me to find the strength I*
>   *need,*
>   *to achieve balance and tranquility.*
> *I ask you to ease my pain dear Lord*
> *And to allow me to release any grief or*
>   *unhappiness*
> *That I may be holding on to.*
> *Help me to love and care for myself,*
> *As you so often care for me.*
> *May I reach out to others for comfort,*
> *And may I also comfort them as I would myself.*
> *I know that I have the strength within me*
> *To easily go beyond any blocks or barriers to*
>   *wellness,*
> *because you have instilled within me the power*

to do so.
Your continued love and Divine guidance are
*   with me always,*
As I find the answers that I have been searching
*   for.*
Amen

Researcher, Masaru Emoto of Japan, discovered that prayer, along with the ingredient of belief can have an effect on molecules of water. If that is the case, then it can ultimately affect our food. His worldwide study of prayer on water showed the difference between water molecules before and after one hour of prayer. Before praying, the water in the photograph appeared to be just a "blob." However after praying near the water, the molecules of water were frozen and the picture revealed a beautifully shaped water crystal. (The photographs of the change in the water molecules can be seen in his books, including the books *The Messages of Water* and *Love Thyself*.)

Remember praying before the meal? In today's hectic society, it can be easy to forget something so simple. But by taking the time to remember where our food came from and feeling grateful for it, we can add to the nourishment that we feel as we enjoy each bite of food that we eat. After all, we instinctively know what and how much food we need. So if we give our troubles to God, the desire to satisfy other needs with food can be released.

The concept of going within our self to heal has been around since ancient times. This ancient wisdom teaches us to connect with ourselves in order to find the answers that we seek. In fact the word "gnosis" (an ancient Greek word) refers to knowledge and insight, or knowledge of the "heart."

When we think of the heart, we think of emotions and the subconscious mind. And when we can tap into those feelings, we can come up with the answers that we seek. It is that divine intuition and inspiration that can help us to discover our own personal needs and desires. Otherwise if we search outside of ourselves, the answers may not be what works for us as a distinct individual.

We can also call it a "transpersonal" approach, which is where the mind, body and spirit are all connected. The belief is that a disconnection from an individual's higher power results in issues on a mental, emotional and physical level. (The transpersonal approach in hypnotherapy helps to re-connect the three to resolve whatever issues an individual may be experiencing.) It is about empowering the individual, by finding the answers within themselves.

Many people feel that divine connection by finding the time to simply meditate. We have so many thoughts going on in our heads while we rush around, searching for answers, but by taking a moment out of our day and quieting the mind, we can reconnect with that feeling of divine peace and serenity.

Rather than staying on the stress "treadmill" with sweets and other foods that are damaging to our health, we can allow ourselves to calm down for a moment so that we can "re-charge." Try turning off the television for a change, and escaping into yourself (because that is where the answers are). In a way, you could say that praying is talking to God, and meditating is listening for the answers.

Connecting with our higher self allows us to have a sense of inner peace and awareness. It is about connecting with our optimal self, and being the best that we can be. What about reading an inspirational book? Perhaps there is someone that you look up to, that may have come a long way in life. Reading his or her story can help you to see that you are capable of attaining whatever goal you desire, but above all, to be in a state of peace and fulfillment. Just open your heart and mind to the possibilities.

Dr. Herbert Benson of Harvard University has his patients use a form of meditation in which he has added prayer. The person chooses a word or phrase that has meaning to them in a religious or philosophical way. By adding this "faith factor," he has improved the effectiveness of the meditation. As a result, the patients have been able to lower their blood pressure and heart rate, and increase muscle relaxation. (To find more information on how to meditate, see the chapter called *Breathe*.)

While you are in a meditative state, be aware that you have access to all of the information that you need to help you. You are able to tap into your own inner wisdom, as well as receive help from any loved ones that may have passed on, or angels, spirit guides, or whomever you may believe is there to assist you.

You can say to yourself "I am connecting with my higher self." See yourself as the loving, empowered being that you are. Notice how you appear to yourself, and remain open to that appearance. While you are in this relaxed, daydream state, ask your higher self (or anyone else that may appear to you such as a loved one) any questions that you would like to be answered. Give yourself time to communicate, and to receive the support and guidance that you need at this time.

When you feel that you have finished, you can thank your higher self (or anyone else that appeared to you) for the information that you received. Keep in mind that you can return to this same state, by placing your thumb and finger together, breathing and relaxing and counting down.

Now that you have completed your time of relaxation and contemplation, start by counting back up from one to five as you slowly become aware of your surroundings. Feelings gradually return to your arms and legs as you reach the number five, and you feel balanced and refreshed when you open your eyes. Even though you are now fully awake and present, you can allow yourself to remember all of the details of the conversation and information you had with either your higher self, or whoever was there to assist you.

Gardening is another way that people feel a connection to the Divine, as plants are part of the earth and can help us to feel "grounded" and connected to the earth. Enjoying plants can be a therapeutic way to feel a connection to another living thing. (Some people even talk to their plants, which they believe helps them to grow and thrive.)

We can also connect to our "universe" and fill whatever emptiness that we may be feeling through service to others. This service could be for people, animals, the earth or whatever inspires us. Replacing food with anything that is positive can fill the void and allow us to shed the excess weight that we may be holding on to.

Harvard psychologist David McClelland conducted research to study the levels of an antibody, called IgA, in students. The level of IgA (which helps the body defend itself against infection) was checked before and after the students watched a film about Mother Teresa, and her work of helping the homeless. It was discovered that the students actually had higher levels of this antibody by simply watching people doing selfless service, which resulted in strengthening their immune system. Proving once again that the mind, body and soul are connected, and they should be treated that way rather than as separate parts.

In the end, diets are simply not the answer. If you stop and think for a moment, how many diets have you tried? How outrageous have they been? Whatever the answer may be, you are not alone. So many other people share the same frustration, as they search for the one diet that will ultimately work. It's time to lose the diet, throw away the scale and focus on ourselves for a change.

And if you must have a diet mantra, then think of these three words: Everything in moderation. In other words, we do not need to deprive ourselves of entire food groups or even certain sweets or "fattening" foods that we love. It's a matter of finding the natural balance that our bodies will automatically go to once we have resolved what is going on "inside" of us. At which time the "outside" will naturally be come balanced, without having to check the numbers on a scale or count calories.

After all, dieting is kind of like going to war with our bodies. If we look at war in our society, what does it really solve? We know that there has to be a better answer, which is to unite with each other and understand that we all come from the same source, whether we call that source "energy" or whatever. In the same way, we must re-connect with ourselves, and in doing so, connect with the source energy that every being is connected to.

We do this by finding our own identity and sense of self, while at the same time giving and receiving support from others. In other words, we must learn to re-connect and be aware of who we really are and by connecting with those around us. By doing so we can feel satisfied, and above all, we can find the inner peace that we naturally crave. As Edgar Cayce said: "Remember, healing — all healing comes from within. Yet there is the healing of the physical, there is the healing of the mental, there is the correct direction from the spirit. Coordinate these and you'll be whole"! Amen to that.

Index

229

Additional copies of *Lose the Diet*
are available through your favorite
book dealer or from the publisher:

Blissful Publications, LLC
3116 S. Mill Avenue #429
Tempe, AZ 85282

www.LoseTheDiet.com

Lose the Diet **(ISBN: 978-0-9821831-0-6)**
is **$19.95** for softbound edition, plus
$5.50 shipping for first copy
($2.00 each additional copy)
and sales tax for **AZ** orders.